Live Well Beyond 120

Here's to a healthy, happy, and meaningful life.

Guy

Live Well Beyond 120

Best Practices for Living a Long, Happy, and Meaningful Life

Gregory Robert Damian

ISBN-13: 978-0-578-69353-8

Cover design by: Mary Ann Demaioribus

Disclaimer

I hope you will find the ideas in this book to be powerful, provocative, and valuable. However, I am not a medical doctor and the material in this book should not be construed as medical advice. The ideas expressed in this book are my opinions, although, wherever possible, I cite references and authorities who are recognized experts in their field. I encourage all readers to discuss with your qualified practitioners the relevance of the application of these ideas to your life.

Table of Contents

Introduction

In my mid-50s, I was listening to a presentation from a spiritual source and I heard the following question: "What is the message that I am sending to the cells of my body?" The question captured my attention and I decided to answer it. My grandmother lived to 100, so my first thoughtful response was "I am going to live to be 105 years old." Upon further reflection, I felt that 105 was not aggressive enough, so I changed my response to "I am going to live to well beyond 120 years."

I lived most of my life without religion and, largely, without spirituality. So, why was I listening to a presentation related to health and beliefs from a spiritual source? Shortly before hearing the presentation, I became open to spirituality entering my life, and new ways of thinking came to me. My new ways of thinking include: we are all one, and the power of belief is missing from the science of longevity.

As I started to share with people close to me that I was going to live well beyond 120, something about what I was saying did not feel right to me. My message felt self-serving and exclusive. With my new beliefs, I came to understand that longevity is not a competition; it is an opportunity for us, collectively, to raise the living experiences of everyone. Knowing that not everyone may choose to or believe that they can live well beyond 120, I decided to assist as many people as possible to live long, happy, and meaningful lives because I know that helping others this way will also help me.

Live Well Beyond 120. Best Practices for Living a Long, Happy, and Meaningful Life is the result of my answering the question of what message I am sending to my cells and is my vehicle for helping other people do the same. The book is based on beliefs, the science of longevity (I cite over 200 sources), and my personal experiences. The list of best practices I created is organized in the categories of Spirit, Body, and Mind.

This is an optimistic book. Even considering the COVID-19 pandemic, I believe that there are many reasons for hope and optimism. I believe, as a species, we will become more cooperative, compassionate, and tolerant and we will develop clean and sustainable ways of living that are beneficial for everyone. We will enter a golden age of peace, prosperity, and of course, longevity.

Acknowledgments

THANK YOU!

I would like to thank Callen Borgias, Tony Borrego, Amy Collette, and Lauren Brombert for encouraging me and giving me feedback during the early development of this book.

I am grateful for Suman Morarka, MD, for her thoughtful feedback of my text.

Several of the articles I reference were brought to my attention by the FUTUREdition e-Newsletter from The Arlington Institute.

I am grateful for the time and effort Mark Chavez, MD, put into helping me develop this book. In addition to providing valuable editing and insights, he showed me how to write more effectively.

I am also grateful for Cory Holly's careful review of my manuscript and showing me several places where I could improve my message.

Lourana Howard, my editor, improved my writing and helped me convey my thoughts more clearly.

I thank Mary Ann Demaioribus, my mother, for helping

me design the cover of this book. The cover photograph was taken by me at Ayampe, Ecuador, March 2018.

I love the clever stick figures from Leremy Gan. I licensed the use of his images from Shutterstock.

I thank early readers of this book who provided important feedback. These readers were: Nina Damian, Mark Damian and Lynn Harms.

I would also like to thank Angela Holloway for supporting and encouraging me to make this the best book possible. Angela is my angel.

Part I. Our Beliefs About Longevity

Your Cells Are Listening

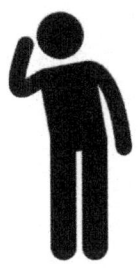

"Your body's cellular structure listens to your consciousness. You can lengthen your lifespan if, daily, you speak to your cellular structure as if it were a workforce for you. You are the boss. What comes out of your mouth is like an order in a restaurant. *You should watch what you say because your cells are listening.*" YCL1

"Your body is aware of your attitude. If you have an attitude that you are nothing and never will be, your body cooperates. Every cell is aware of your attitude." YCL2

These messages from Kryon, delivered through Lee Carroll, inspired this book. Carroll started getting loving, hopeful, and optimistic messages from an entity he calls Kryon in 1989. These messages shocked him. He was an engineer and had no interest in anything metaphysical or esoteric. I started listening to Kryon's messages after my own spiritual awakening, which I describe later.

Kryon discusses the blending of science and spirituality, with human consciousness being the linkage. Kryon says that, with our consciousness, we "can change how fast and how profoundly our body ages." We can instruct our cells to "age slower," by telling our cells to "age only every other day." Kryon emphasizes that we need to give our cells instructions every day. In the absence of specific instructions, our cells listen to the messages of our culture, such as we get old and die at a certain age.

Carrol says science is beginning to call the linkage between science and spirituality epigenetics. I studied mechanical and biomedical engineering. As an engineer, this blending of science and spirituality is important to me.

After I heard the "your cells are listening" messages from Kryon, I heard similar messages from other spiritual leaders. In a talk given by Wayne Dyer titled, "Stop Wasting Time and Start Greatness, Turn Your No-Limit Person from Zero to Hero," Dyer said, what happens to our cells is a result of the way we think. In *Conversations with God, Book 4: Awaken the Species*, Neale Donald Walsch wrote, "You are right if you are suggesting that the energy of your thoughts has an influence over the cells of your body." YCL3

The question of what instructions I should send to my cells captured my attention and I decided to answer it. My grandmother lived to 100, so my first thoughtful response was "I am going to live to be 105 years old."

How Long We Live

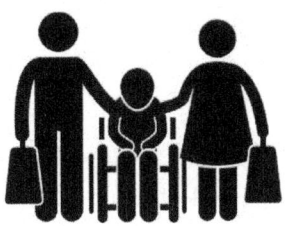

How reasonable is it for me or anyone else to expect to live to 105 years of age?

According to the Center for Disease Control, as of 2017, the life expectancy for all people in the United States is 78.6 years. For men, life expectancy is 76.1 years and for women, life expectancy is 81.1 years. In the U.S., Hispanic women's life expectancy is 84.3 years, while black men have the lowest life expectancy of 71.9 years.[HLL1] Worldwide, the tiny European country of Monaco has the longest average life expectancy of 89.5 years, while Chad only has a life expectancy of 49.8 years.[HLL2] Several other African countries have life expectancies of less than 55 years.

Because of the unreliability of old birth records, the age of the longest living modern man and woman is not clear. There is a report of a man in Bolivia, Carmelo Flores Laura, who lived to 123 years of age.[HLL3] The Gerontology Research Group lists the longest living male, with proper documentation, as Masazou Nonaka from Japan, who lived 113.5 years.[HLL4] They list the longest living female as Nabi Tajima, also from Japan, who lived 117.7 years. Guinness World Records reports the oldest verified person was Jeanne Calment of France, who died in 1997. She was 122.4 years of age when she passed.

The first book of the Bible suggests that humans lived much longer than we do today. The website, "Answers in Genesis," indicates several biblical characters lived to be over 900 years old.[HLL5] There is no way to validate these figures. However, *Conversations With God: An Uncommon Dialogue, Book 1*, says, "Do you really think the best God could do was a body that could make it 60, 70, maybe 80 years before falling apart? Is that, do you imagine, the limit of My ability?... I designed your magnificent body to last forever!" [HLL6]

Longevity is a part of my heritage. My maternal grandmother, Gertrude Cecilia Weber, lived to be 100.[HLL7] My grandmother had several sisters that lived into their 90s and beyond as well. My maternal great-grandmother, Nettie Franz Weber, was born in 1879 and lived to be 91. My mother is a young and healthy 78 and has the potential to live at least as long as her mother. My father made little effort to take care of himself and, despite this, lived 82 years. My paternal grandfather lived to be 91, although my paternal grandmother died relatively young from complications from diabetes.

Many longevity predictors and calculators are easily accessible on the web. You enter a few details about yourself and the calculator will tell you how long you can expect to live. The Social Security Administration's Life Expectancy Calculator needs a few simple inputs. It predicts that I will live another 26 years, to age 83.[HLL8] I took the BLUE ZONES® True Vitality Test as well.[HLL9] This short assessment of risk factors is based on the BLUE ZONES® research which I will discuss later. My results indicate I should live to be 94.4 years. The assessment also indicated I could live an additional 2.7 years through various lifestyle modifications.

In addition, you can assess your current biological age through a series of questions evaluating your habits related to diet, exercise, objective measurements such as blood pressure, smoking, drinking, stress, and fulfillment. One such assessment is RealAge®, offered through *Sharecare.com*. I took the assessment when I was 57 years and 4 months old and my RealAge® was 49 years and 6 months.

After a few weeks of sending the message of "I am going to live to be 105 years of age" to my cells, the thought occurred to me that living to 105 was not aggressive enough, so I changed my beliefs and instructions to 120 years. Additionally, I added "well beyond" resulting in, "I am going to live well beyond 120 years." "Well beyond" has two meanings. The first meaning is that these are going to be high-quality years, years with happiness and purpose. The second meaning is that I will live at least, but not limited to, 120 years.

Our Beliefs About Health and Longevity

Our beliefs about health and longevity are powerful. The placebo effect is one example that is well documented, though still not completely accepted by western medicine. The Oxford Dictionary defines the placebo effect as "a beneficial effect produced by a placebo drug or treatment, which cannot be attributed to the properties of the placebo itself, and must, therefore, be due to the patient's belief in that treatment."

Ted Kaptchuk, of Harvard Medical School, who focuses on the placebo effect, says people associate taking medicine with a positive healing effect.[BAL1] Just the action of taking a pill, real or not, can stimulate the brain into thinking the body is being healed. He also says we can induce our own placebo effect by "engaging in the ritual of healthy living – eating right, exercising, yoga, quality social time, and meditating."

Since beliefs can bias both patients and study administrators, clinical studies must be conducted in a "double-blind" fashion to attempt to remove beliefs and biases. Double-blind studies divide the subjects into two groups. One group receives the drug and the other group receives a pill (placebo) that looks exactly like the drug but has none of the active compounds being tested.

The administrators of the treatments are not permitted to know which subjects are receiving the drug or the placebo or they could influence the subjects and the outcomes. This is what makes the study double-blind. The researchers look at the outcomes from the group who received the drug compared with the group who received the placebo. The challenge for the researchers is that the placebo effect may account for much of the drug's effect.[BAL2] Faith Brynie, PhD, in her article published in *Psychology Today*, reports, "Estimates of the placebo cure rate range from a low of 15% to a high of 72%." [BAL3]

Here are a few common unhealthy beliefs related to longevity.

"I am afraid of growing old because that means I will be weak and frail."

"Human lifespan has peaked. A barrier has been reached."

"Age is a good predictor of when you'll die."

"The longer you live, the harder it is to change and adapt."

"When I get old, I will not be able to take care of myself."

"Getting old means the death of friends and relatives. I will be lonely."

> "I may not be able to work and if I still can, I will
> be considered slow, old-fashioned, and unable to
> keep up with younger workers."

> "By the time I reach 75, I will have lived a
> complete life."

"By the time I reach 75, I will have lived a complete life,"
is a quote by Ezekiel Emanuel from his 2014 Atlantic
article titled, "Why I hope to die at 75." [BAL4] Emanuel
lays out his case for why 75 years of living will be
enough for him. I appreciate that he has a plan for his
living days and is looking to make the most of them. I
have no doubt that Emanuel's wishes will be granted to
him, but I believe we can do better than that.

"How do we stop and reverse the aging process?" Esther
Hicks, an inspirational speaker and author, was asked
this question in one of her question-and-answer sessions.
Her response was that the words "aging process" exhibit
belief in inevitable decline and the belief in decline is
responsible for the aging process. It is also this belief that
will not allow for a reversing of the aging process.

The "Fear of Getting Old" webpage offered its readers a
survey asking, "How afraid of getting old are you?" [BAL5]
81% of respondents selected "Somewhat Afraid" or
"Very Afraid." My immediate thought was this must be
a survey of older people. However, I learned that 45% of
the respondents were under 18 years of age, and 44%
were between 19 and 34 years. This is fear of aging in

younger people. Of course, this is not a representative sample of the entire population of young people. Someone who visits a web page about the fear of getting old probably has beliefs that would lead them to that page.

In 2013, Pew Research conducted several polls related to beliefs of longevity.[BAL6] The surveys included results from over 2,000 nationally representative U.S. adults from all 50 states. The margin of error is declared to be plus or minus 2.9%.

In the Pew survey, 25% of U.S. adults say that, by 2050, the average person in the U.S. will definitely or probably live to be at least 120 years old. 73% of respondents said this definitely or probably will not happen. When asked how long they would like to live, 8% of people cite an age of greater than 100. 69% cite an age between 79 and 100. The median ideal lifespan in the survey was 90 years. 90 years was about 11 years longer than the 2013 average U.S. life expectancy. Overall, about 41% of U.S. adults consider the growing number of elderly people in the population to be a good thing for society. Only 10% of those surveyed thought more older people would be bad for society. 61% indicated the growing world population will be a major problem because there may not be enough food and resources.

What beliefs do you have about aging? Do you believe your longevity is determined by your genes?

Adult height is out of our control and height has been found to be inversely correlated with longevity.[BAL7] This means that, other things being equal, shorter people tend to live longer than taller people. Does this mean taller people cannot live well beyond 120? I do not believe that is the case.

A 1995 study of Danish twins looked to determine the impact of genetics on longevity.[BAL8] This study involved 2,872 twin pairs who survived to at least the age of 15. The study concluded that longevity seems to be only "moderately inheritable." The study estimated the overall inheritability of longevity as 26% for males and 23% for females. The gender differences were caused by the "impact of non-shared environmental factors," typically, the work environment.

I propose that genetics does not determine your longevity unless you believe it does.

Living 120 Years Is Like Running a Four-Minute Mile

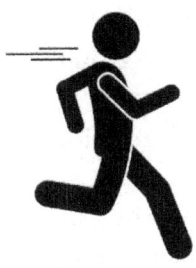

Once Roger Bannister broke the four-minute-mile running barrier, many other runners also broke the barrier. Once the 120-year barrier is broken, many more people will choose and experience this and it will become a new normal.

Some researchers are on board. Bryan G. Hughes and Siegfried Hekimi, in a study published in *Nature* in 2017, state there is "no detectable limit to how long people can live." FMM1

Certainly, not everyone believes humans can live longer than we currently do. Some people believe we are "done" and nothing further is possible. Mark, et al., in their article published in *Frontiers in Physiology* in 2017, asked, "Are We Reaching the Limits of Homo Sapiens?" FMM2 Unlike Hughes and Hekimi, Mark and his colleagues propose that we are already at our biological limits. The authors point to plateauing athletic performance in track and field events as evidence that we, as a species, are not only plateauing but are at risk of regressing. The authors state, "When plateaus are reached, care should then be taken to prevent regression, even if remaining close to the upper limits may become more costly." The authors cite limited ability for adaptation and environmental deterioration as reasons for plateauing. Indeed, these are powerful beliefs, and I believe they are only limitations if we allow them to be.

Not everyone can run a four-minute mile. Anyone who aspires to run that fast has to do several things. They must train correctly and have the proper nutrition and rest. A one-mile running event happens quickly, but training for it takes years.

My best time for a mile was just over five minutes. I was quite surprised to learn that I could run a mile in under six minutes. Could I have run a mile in under four minutes? I do not know. In hindsight, I believe I could have run in under five minutes for a mile had I set my intention to do it. I am clear that, in my 50s, a four-minute mile is not possible and so, that is my reality.

I propose that living well beyond 120 years is a barrier of beliefs and will require intention and good practices.

Research That Influenced My Knowledge and Beliefs About Longevity

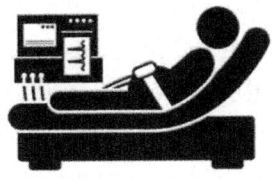

The research in this chapter influenced my knowledge and beliefs about longevity. I believe this is important to share because, in addition to beliefs, I want to apply the best strategies that science can offer. Some people may have enough faith to overcome a terrible diet and a sedentary lifestyle, but most faith is not that strong.

I was trained as a mechanical engineer and worked as a technology project manager. However, in 2004, I left my job because I wanted to go to medical school. This was a bold move as I was already in my 40s. I took the prerequisite biology and chemistry courses and studied for, took, and scored well on the challenging Medical College Admissions Test. Along the way, I realized that I was really interested in natural approaches to health and longevity. So, rather than go to medical school, I decided to study biomedical engineering with the possibility of earning a PhD degree. Unfortunately, my sponsor's research was related to the mechanical properties of DNA and this had nothing to do with longevity, so I returned to my prior work. These studies, however, provided me with the educational background to better understand the science related to health and longevity.

Also, in 2004, I read Roy Wofford, MD's book, *The 120-Year Diet: How to Double Your Vital Years.*[RBL1] Dr. Wofford was the physician in the first mission of Biosphere II. Set in rural Arizona, the project was an experiment to determine the viability of a closed ecosystem to sustain human life. The project was inspired by requirements of long-term space missions, such as going to Mars. The small team of people had to grow all of their own food but found it difficult to supply themselves with enough calories. "Over a two-year period ... crops failed, resulting in the restriction of the occupants' diets to 1,750 calories per day." [RBL2] The participants were slowly starving themselves to death.

Dr. Wofford observed that even though the participants, himself included, were starving, they were relatively healthy. After the project ended, Dr. Wofford went on to promote the concept of calorie restriction to increase longevity. Calorie restriction has been shown in the laboratory to lengthen the lifespan of small mammals, such as mice.[RBL3] Humans live much longer lives than mice, so it has not been possible to prove that severe calorie restriction would work in the case of humans, if they were willing to implement the regimen. It is interesting to note that the older mice did not respond as well to calorie restriction as younger mice, which might have implications for humans.

Research That Influenced My Knowledge and Beliefs About Longevity

Calorie restriction gave scientists an avenue to explore the physiology of life extension.[RBL4] They looked for chemical compounds that could potentially induce the same biological responses of calorie restriction without having to endure the calorie restriction protocol. Resveratrol has been identified as a possible compound and has been studied in this regard. While it is far from proven that resveratrol lengthens the lifespan of humans, several potential benefits of resveratrol have been identified, including lowering blood pressure, protecting the brain, improving insulin sensitivity, and easing joint pain.[RBL5]

Besides resveratrol, other longevity-promoting compounds being investigated include metformin, rapamycin, and nicotinamide mononucleotide (NMN). In the U.S., metformin and rapamycin are prescription drugs though not approved by the FDA as anti-aging therapies. Resveratrol, NMN, and the related nicotinamide riboside (NR) are sold as over-the-counter supplements.

There is enthusiasm related to NMN and NR. They are both forms of vitamin B and have been shown to reverse vascular aging in mice.[RBL6] We need to be careful before we get too excited. There were early concerns that rapamycin might cause cancer [RBL7], but these fears have not been realized. Just the opposite appears to be the case as one study found that rapamycin can extend life by preventing cancer.[RBL8]

In Suzanne Somers' book, *Bombshell*,[RBL9] she lays out 18 factors associated with aging and offers a supplement strategy to address each. The aging factors she lists are:

Chronic Inflammation – an immune response that does not subside;

Glycation – sugars binding to proteins or fats, forming unnatural structures;

Methylation – a reduction of the methylation processes that protect and repair damaged DNA;

Mitochondrial dysfunction – mitochondria, organelles that are responsible for the production of energy units of ATP, degrade over time;

Loss of mitochondria – In addition to mitochondrial dysfunction, the number of mitochondria diminish over time;

Hormone imbalance – natural production of some hormones decline over time and create imbalances;

Excess calcification – calcification of cells of the heart valves and brain;

Digestive enzyme deficit – enzymes necessary for digestion decline as we age;

Fatty acid imbalance – imbalances of essential fatty acids;

DNA mutation – exposure to carcinogens and toxins damage our DNA and, over time, our body loses its ability to repair the damage;

Immune dysfunction – there is a reduced level of immune response over time;

Enzyme imbalance – detrimental enzyme imbalances in the brain and liver resulting in neurological damage;

Excitotoxicity – damage to nerve cells due to excessive stimulation from neurotransmitters;

Circulatory deficit – lack of blood flow to organs due to endothelial dysfunction;

Loss of youthful gene expression – genes that maintain cellular health shut down;

Insulin sensitivity – aging reduces insulin sensitivity;

Loss of bone density – the gradual loss of bone density; and

Oxidative stress – cellular damage due to free radicals.

The above list does not include the supplements that Somers recommends for each of the factors of aging. However, the Life Extension Foundation article reviewing her book noted that fish oil, vitamin D, lipoic acid, curcumin, CoQ10, resveratrol, DHEA, vitamin K, and SAMe occur repeatedly in her recommendations and have multiple benefits. The article suggests that everyone interested in longevity consider these supplements.[RBL10]

Dan Buettner sought out and studied areas around the planet where people lived the longest. His work resulted in the book called, *The Blue Zones: 9 Lessons for Living Longer From the People Who've Lived the Longest*.[RBL11] He studied people in the following areas: the Greek island, Icaria; the Barbagia region of Sardinia; Okinawa Japan;

the Nicoya peninsula of Costa Rica; and the Seventh-day Adventists in Loma Linda, California. In studying these exceptionally long-lived people, Buettner and his team came up with nine common behaviors that they associated with longevity.

> **Move Naturally** – The world's longest-lived people move without thinking about it. They walk. They work in gardens.
>
> **Purpose** – The study says that "knowing your sense of purpose is worth up to seven years of extra life expectancy."
>
> **Down Shift** – The studied people manage their stress with meditation, prayer, and rest.
>
> **80% Rule** – The study observed that people stop eating before feeling full.
>
> **Plant Slant** – Plant-based diets are normal for these people.
>
> **Wine @ 5** – People in the studied groups, except the Seventh-day Adventists, drink alcohol regularly, moderately, and do not abuse it.
>
> **Belong to Some Faith-based System** – It does not matter which faith system.
>
> **Loved Ones First** – The studied people are family-centric. They tend to live with or close to their family members.
>
> **Right Tribe** – The world's longest-lived people have healthy social communities.

A recently-published study of 17,660 Chinese people, who were over 80 years of age, confirms most, but not all, of the BLUE ZONES® findings.[RBL12] This study found that "never smoking, never drinking, physical exercise, ideal diet, and normal weight were associated with lower mortality." Further, the study found that "former and current smoking, former drinking, never exercising, and (being) underweight were associated with increased mortality." This study also looked at whether the potentially harmful effect of risk factors could be counteracted by a healthy lifestyle in these subjects. The answer was yes. "Our findings further confirm the efficacy of an integrated approach to healthy longevity, which considers various lifestyle practices in conjunction (as opposed to in isolation) among the oldest-old. Our results emphasize the value of promoting healthy living as a preventive strategy, and to improve the management of healthy lifestyles."

What is common from Roy Wofford's work, the BLUE ZONES® research, and the Chinese study are diet, exercise, and lifestyle practices which include faith, prayer and meditation, minimizing stress, having purpose, and a supportive community. In addition, there is reason to consider supplements and compounds such as resveratrol and fish oil as a part of a comprehensive strategy for longevity.

My Spiritual Transformation

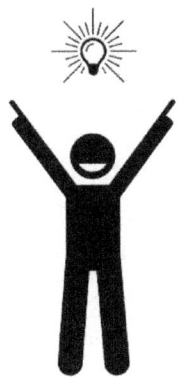

Because of my spiritual transformation, this book is possible. Even though I was aware and knowledgeable of longevity before my transformation, my new spirituality is influencing my thoughts and recommendations about longevity in many important ways.

I was raised by Catholic parents, and I completed the Catholic tradition of confirmation. However, the practice of rituals and a judgmental God never made sense to me, so I left the Catholic church after I graduated from high school. After leaving the church, I studied the Greek text of the Bible in an attempt to find the true meaning of the Scriptures. I did not feel moved or inspired by this, and it still seemed like the interpretation was largely dependent upon the individual doing the interpreting. This would have been fine, had I agreed with the interpretation. I tried other Christian churches, but none of them resonated with me. For the next 30 years, I embraced science and materialism. I was indifferent to religion and spirituality, with one exception: the music and lyrics of the band, Kansas. Many of the songs written by Kerry Livgren, including "Dust In The Wind" and "The Wall" had spiritual messages that I related to.

In a self-improvement class I took in 2015, I performed an exercise where we were paired with a buddy. We had to give our buddy a gift that represented something that we did not see in ourselves. In my case, my buddy was giving me a gift related to spirituality. I said to myself, "Oh great, here comes a Bible." Instead, the gift my buddy gave me was a small statue of a Hindu goddess. It was perfect for me because I realized how narrowly I had been perceiving spirituality. It had never occurred to me there were forms of spirituality other than the ones I had been previously exposed to. I did not adopt Hinduism, but the doors of new possibilities were now open for me.

About a year after that exercise, I met a very special woman. Her name is Angela and she is an angel. After several months of dating (I had been divorced a year earlier), she innocently handed me the book, *Conversations with God: An Uncommon Dialogue, Book 1* (CWG), written by Neale Donald Walsch.[MST1] She said that she had read the book several years ago and it changed her way of thinking about God and spirituality. Had she been dogmatic or demanding in her approach, I surely would have pushed the book away. I started reading the book and could not put it down.

In the mid-1990s, Walsch wrote a series of books that were transcripts of the "conversations" that he had with God. Walsch was also raised Catholic, and Walsch's own process led him to seek teachings beyond the Catholic faith. At the point in his life where he started having conversations with God, he had been homeless for a year. He decided to write a letter to God with "a pile of angry questions." Much to his surprise, he received answers. "Do you really want an answer to all these questions, or are you just venting?" Walsch responded that he did want answers and began a dialog that produced ten books containing over 3,000 pages of information.

I was fascinated by *Conversations With God* and the subsequent CWG books. The material made sense to me. I have read and listened to each of the books more than 12 times. Prior to reading these books, I had never read a book more than once. Rather than just reading, I was studying, although I was not sure why.

I learned the three fundamental principles of CWG:

> We are all one.
> There is enough.
> There is nothing you have to do.

The first statement, "We are all one," is profound and has meaning well beyond this simple statement. This is completely consistent with what Jesus said, "Do unto others as you would have them do unto you." MST2 This is also known as the Golden Rule. I believe our success as a species is completely dependent upon our cooperation with each other.

CWG encourages us to think, create, and experience the life that we choose. Like most spiritual systems that I am aware of, CWG fully embraces the concept of free will. CWG wants us to find our own truth. Disagreeing with the CWG material is encouraged. We do not have to be limited by others' beliefs or fear that our choices will condemn us. Kryon agrees. Kryon says that God would not give us free will only to punish us if we make the "wrong" choice. This, of course, does not mean that our choices are free from earthly consequences or outcomes of physical laws.

It is not the intention of CWG to create a new religion, but rather, to enhance, complete, or fulfill the existing religions and belief systems on the planet. CWG makes this statement to emphasize the point: "Ours is not a better way. Ours is simply another way."

CWG makes several observations related to human health:

> "I hate to suggest this because it sounds so mundane coming from God, but – for God's sake, take better care of yourself."

> "You do not exercise your body, so it grows flabby and, worse yet, weak from non-use."

"You do not nourish your body properly, thereby weakening it further. Then you fill it with toxins and poisons and the most absurd substances posing as food."

"You fail to prevent breakdowns with regular checkups, once-a-year physicals, and to use the therapies and medicines you've been given."

"The conditions under which you ask your body to survive are horrible. But you will do little or nothing about them. You will read this, nod your head in regretful agreement, and go right back to the mistreatment. And do you know why? Because you have *no will to live*."

"Everything depends on who you think you are, and what you are trying to do. If your objective is to live a life of good health and great longevity, consuming dead flesh, smoking known carcinogens, and drinking volumes of nerve-deadening, brain-frying liquids do not work."

"An illness is created first in the mind. Worry, hate, fear – together with their offshoots: anxiety, bitterness, impatience, avarice, unkindness, judgmentalness, and condemnation – all attack the body at the cellular level. It is impossible to have a healthy body under these conditions."

I met Neale Donald Walsch personally in July of 2018. He came to Denver for a three-day seminar in support of his latest book, *Conversations With God, Book 4, Awaken the Species*.[MST3] There were a number of people present who were as familiar with the CWG material as I was, and I enjoyed listening to Walsch speak live and interacting with all of the attendees.

I found Lee Carroll after I was introduced to Walsch's books. I have attended three Kryon presentations.

In the summer of 2019, I attempted to have my own conversations with God in a similar fashion to Neale Donald Walsch. I would wake up in the middle of the night and ask God questions. I did get a lot of answers, but in retrospect, these answers were summaries of the material of CWG. I do not believe that I received new revelations the way Walsch did.

When I became willing to accept that something else was possible, my life changed.

We Are All In This Together

Perhaps my claim of living well beyond 120 is still too timid. Perhaps, we can live forever. In another way, my statement of living to at least 120 is unusual and provocative. Normally, people do not declare how long they are going to live. One exception is actor Sterling K. Brown, who, at 43, said he plans to live to 100.[ALL1] Another exception is Suzanne Somers, who, in 2009, when she was 62 years old and after surviving breast cancer, shared that "I'm going to live for 110 years." [ALL2] There is also David Sinclair, PhD, an Australian, who is one of the world's leading researchers on aging. He recently published a book titled, *Lifespan: Why We Age – and Why We Don't Have To*. In the article, *The End of Aging*, Chris Taylor quotes Dr. Sinclair as saying he would like to see the turn of the next century, which would make him 132 years old.[ALL3]

Why don't more people declare in advance how long they are going to live? One can argue, "we just do not know." Obviously, there are, or appear to be, circumstances beyond our control that can terminate our physical lives. We can be in the wrong place at the wrong time. Other people take a more passive approach of "que sera sera" – what will be will be. Further, it might appear boastful or selfish to declare that one is going to live to an advanced age. We are also obsessed, in our culture, with being right. No one wants to be wrong. I am willing to be wrong.

If I am right, I will not be alone. The population of people living to be at least 100, known as centenarians, is growing rapidly. The United Nations Department of Economic and Social Affairs reported, "The number of centenarians will grow … from less than 343,000 in 2012 to 3.2 million in 2050." ALL4

It is one thing for me to have a private belief about how long I am going to live. However, it is another thing altogether for me to tell people about it. As I started to share with people close to me that I was going to live well beyond 120, something about what I was saying did not feel right to me. My message felt self-serving and exclusive.

The idea that a small number of people should benefit from longevity strategies, while the quality of life for many people is still quite low, is, at least, selfish and is a tragedy for people experiencing poverty. This tragedy is even more acute when it is driven by a lack of will rather than a lack of resources. For example, there is plenty of food and water, but we, as a race, choose not to distribute it to all of the places where it is needed.

I believe every single person on the planet is equally special and important. No one is better than anyone else. Not rich people or poor people, not white people or people of color, not democrats or republicans, not educated people or illiterate people, not healthy people or sick people. We can and must improve the opportunity for every single person because we are all one.

While I was considering this, I read Pagan Kennedy's article, "The Secret to a Longer Life? Don't Ask These Dead Longevity Researchers." ALL5 In the article, Kennedy made two profound statements that resonated with me. "We should all fight for other people's health. Your decisions can affect me when I die and vice versa," and "Aging is not some kind of competitive sport you play against your peers. When it comes to staying alive, we're all in it together." In this article, Kennedy interviewed Dr. Charles Brenner, who in 2004 discovered the cellular effects of NR agreed, saying, "*the decisions that we make collectively might be the most important ones.*"

The quotes from the article reminded me of the CWG quote, "*That which you wish to experience for yourself, cause another to experience.*" Knowing that not everyone may choose to or believe that they can live well beyond 120, I decided to assist as many people as possible to live long, happy and meaningful lives. Further, I pledge at least one-third of the profits from this book and any related speaking, teaching, or coaching to improve basic living conditions for people living in poverty.

I am excited to help people live long, happy and meaningful lives!

Part II. Longevity Best Practices Based on Beliefs, Science, and My Experience

If our "cells are listening," why is belief not enough? Perhaps it is, but we see aging and death all around us. We have a death and dying culture. As long as we feel that early death is a natural way of life, then we need to pay attention to the practices that bring forth the best health possible.

Based on beliefs, scientific research, and my experience, I created a list of best practices to not only live longer but also to have a happy and meaningful life. These best practices are organized in categories of Spirit, Body, and Mind. Many books have been written about each one of these topics. I am going to briefly describe and elaborate on each best practice, bringing forward what I believe is special and interesting from scientific and personal perspectives.

My first spirit-based longevity best practice is about having positive beliefs of longevity and yourself. The idea of beliefs comes through again and again in several of the other best practices. I discuss having a faith-based or spiritual practice and praying or meditating. It is clear to me that having a purpose in life and being service-oriented is vital. Without relationships with other people and animals, most of us would not have meaning in our lives. I discuss the importance of being happy and present. Finally, aesthetics, how we look and feel about ourselves, is included in this section because it affects how long we live.

My body-based longevity best practices include eating a natural diet, moving your body, and having a health plan. In addition, I discuss supplements, body composition, and hormone management. The final recommendation is to avoid substances that can do our bodies harm. In the group of mind-based longevity best practices, I discuss strategies for protecting the brain, minimizing stress, and getting the proper amount of sleep.

Spirit-Based Longevity Best Practices

Have Positive Beliefs of Longevity
Have a Faith or Spiritual Practice
Pray or Meditate
Have Healthy Relationships
Be Purposeful and Service-Oriented
Be Happy and Present
Use Aesthetics to Feel Better and Live Longer

Have Positive Beliefs of Longevity

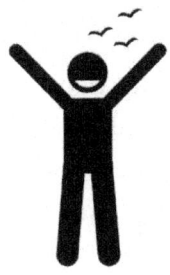

The best practices begin with having positive beliefs of life and longevity. In the earlier chapter, "Our Beliefs About Health and Longevity," I discussed many beliefs we have about our health and longevity and the power of those beliefs. Mahatma Gandhi's quote summarizes it well, "*when I believe I can, then I acquire the ability to do it even if I didn't have it in the beginning.*"

Since our beliefs are powerful and they drive every thought and behavior in our life, we would be wise to understand what our beliefs are and where our they come from.

Our beliefs begin forming when we are quite young. The article, "Transforming the Workforce for Children Birth Through Age 8," states,

> "From very early on, children are not simply passive observers, registering the superficial appearance of things. Rather, they are building explanatory systems — implicit theories — that organize their knowledge. These theories enable children to predict, explain, and reason about

relevant phenomena and, in some cases, intervene to change them. As early as the first year of life, babies are developing theories about how the world of people, other living things, objects, and numbers operates. It is important to point out that these foundational theories are not simply isolated forms of knowledge, but play a profound role in children's everyday lives and subsequent education." [PBL1]

Beliefs formed as young people become the basis of beliefs for the rest of our lives. While healthy for an eight-year-old, these beliefs are not necessarily healthy for an adult. Unfortunately, we are generally not aware of our beliefs.

A belief inventory is a tool used to understand our beliefs. Abigail Brenner, MD, who wrote the article for *Psychology Today* titled, "The Belief Inventory," says the belief inventory describes who you are at this point in time and will help you clarify what you believe.[PBL2] Belief inventories usually cover all aspects of one's life, including personal, professional, and social. In her article, Brenner suggests several questions to ask yourself about your beliefs, including:

> What are the beliefs you know in your heart to be true?

> What are the beliefs that others have about you that are or are not true?

Do you have fear about being in a relationship? Why?

Do you have secrets that you never want to be revealed? What would happen if they were revealed?

What are the skills or gifts that are expressed in your work?

What creative aspects of yourself have you never pursued or expressed?

What are your religious or spiritual beliefs? How do these beliefs serve or represent you?

The level of introspection necessary to create a belief inventory is high. It is not typically something that one can do in an hour. It may take several observations of your thoughts and behaviors to begin the process of understanding your core beliefs. Dr. Bruce Lipton, PhD, says if you have any doubt about your beliefs, look at your life. "Your life is a blueprint of your subconscious programming."

There are tests that you can take to determine your biases, subconscious forms of belief. The Implicit Association Test (IAT) from Harvard is one such test.[PBL3] When I took the test, it revealed biases in race and religion, even when I felt that I was neutral.

Dr. Brenner instructs us, "What you believe is not written in stone and can be altered to better fit who you are within a specific stage or life circumstance." Once we have awareness of beliefs and biases that do not serve us, we can start making small changes that can lead to larger changes.

When Mahzarin Banaji, one of the founders of the IAT and co-author of the book *Blindspot: Hidden Biases of Good People*, took her own racial bias test, she reported she was embarrassed by her results.[PBL4] She took action by posting pictures of successful people of color in her office to reprogram her brain and to reinforce her desired belief that all people are good.

Being present, repetition, and positive affirmations reinforce changes in behaviors we want to make. Here are several positive affirmations that I use every day:

Something amazing is happening to us.

I am love and I am loved.

We are love and we are loved.

Every day and every way, I am becoming kinder.

I believe that I am worthy of helping other people live long, happy, and meaningful lives. Here are some affirmations I use to reinforce this belief:

I am grateful for my amazing and healthy body.

Our health comes from our collective actions.

My cells age every other day.

My immune system was designed for this moment and is stronger than it has ever been.

I am helping other people live long, happy, and meaningful lives.

What underlying beliefs drive you? What action would help you change a belief that does not serve or represent you? Do you believe you are capable or worthy of living a long, happy, and meaningful life? What messages and attitudes are you sending to your cells?

"What you think is who you are. What you expect, you become. What you want, you can manifest." Kryon.

Have a Faith or Spiritual Practice

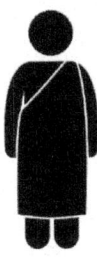

Having a faith-based or spiritual practice can add years to our lives. In a sample of people from Des Moines, Iowa, those people affiliated with a religious practice lived 9.4 years longer than those not affiliated. In a larger sample of people across 42 U.S. cities, the religiously affiliated lived 5.6 years longer than the nonaffiliated.[FSP1] The authors of these studies discussed why they believed they found a positive correlation between affiliation with a religious organization and longevity, and provided these explanations: social support that comes with being a part of a group, caring and service for others, stress reduction, and positive self-esteem leading to other healthy behaviors.

The research did not investigate if one faith-based practice is more effective than another, and I am not here to tell you what to believe. Your path is whatever it is, and it is perfect for you.

Earlier in this book, I shared with you my path to spirituality because it has been essential for me in delivering this information to you.

I have joined a church in Denver and have been attending regularly. I relate to the guiding principles of the church which are:

We believe in God.

We believe God is in everyone and in everything.

We believe God is Love.

We believe we are spiritual beings in a material existence.

We believe we create our own reality with our thoughts.

We believe we are here in this physical world to learn and to develop our spirituality.

We believe it is our responsibility to continue to develop and perfect our character throughout our lives.

We believe God has spoken to us through many teachers throughout history.

We believe the Gifts of Spirit are given to us by God.

We believe each of us is a cell in the body of God. We believe in Endless Possibilities and the Power of Faith.

I emphasize that the above list is *not* what you have to believe. This list represents many of my truths, at least for now. In addition to this church, I also appreciate the teachings of the Unity Church and have attended several Hindu workshops and services. I found Paramahansa Yogananda's *Autobiography of a Yogi* a delightful read.

I do not have any animosity toward any belief system. I have been able to reconcile my differences with the Catholic Church. In fact, I am a fan of some of the statements that Pope Francis has made. In particular, I was impressed by the statement he made to the small number of Catholics in Morocco. He said, "their mission was not to convert their neighbors but to live in brotherhood with other faiths." FSP2 He went on to say, "The Church grows not through proselytism but by attraction."

Through my church, I have taken Reiki (energy work) training and am a Reiki Master. There have been studies related to the effectiveness of Reiki and other "energy" healing modalities. Bernard Grad pioneered the study of energy work. "In carefully controlled experiments, Grad found that selected healers could influence the germination of plant seeds, the growth rate of plants, and the curing of seeds that had been shocked by a saline solution. In addition, he was able to measure the ability of healers to reduce goiter and stimulate wound healing in mice." FSP3

I have a few suggestions if you currently do not have a faith or spiritual practice.

Define your truth.

Set the intention of what you are looking for. Ask for it.

Be open to having different experiences from what you might be expecting.

Follow your intuition and your heart.

Be patient. It takes time to develop spiritual beliefs, community, and relationships.

Consider what you can contribute and do not just selfishly seek the benefits you can derive. I have found that bringing value to someone else will accelerate your experience.

Minimize your judgments to allow you to see the perfection in whatever you are doing.

Be tolerant of the practices and beliefs of others.

Have no expectations of other people and do not require others to believe what you believe.

I believe that the path to peace on our planet is to be tolerant of the practices and beliefs of others.

Pray or Meditate

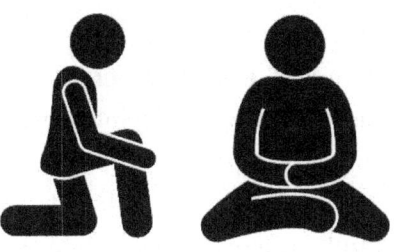

Prayer and meditation are ancient practices dating back thousands of years, and there is a large body of knowledge related to prayer and meditation, including how to pray or meditate, and the benefits of prayer and meditation.[POM1]

I have heard it said that prayer is talking to God and meditation is listening. The Billy Graham Association sees prayer as a two-way spiritual communication between an individual and God, in which an individual not only talks to God but also listens.[POM2] The website and publication, *Healthline*, describes meditation as "a habitual process of training your mind to focus and redirect your thoughts."[POM3]

There are many benefits reported from prayer and meditation.[POM4, POM5] Here are just a few:

> Reduced stress
> Reduced anxiety
> Lengthened attention span
> Reduced age-related memory loss
> Improved sleep

Reduced pain
Improved blood pressure
Improved heart and respiratory rates
Improved cholesterol levels
Increased feelings of social connection

In many 12-step programs, the 11th step starts with, "Sought through prayer and meditation to improve our conscious contact with God as we understood God." POM6 *Recovery.org* describes the purpose of the 11th step as helpful for creating "a solid foundation for a peaceful and fulfilled life and to develop a more positive way of thinking, which will better serve you moving forward." POM7

The good news, according to *WebMD.com*, is that only 10 minutes of daily meditation is needed to begin to see benefits.POM8

In an article on the website, *PrayerOnline.org*, Tricia McCary Rhodes describes several types of prayer including:POM9

> **Intercession**. Intercessory prayer means praying earnestly for the needs of others;
> **Supplication**. Supplication prayer petitions someone for something;
> **Faith**. To ask for what is promised in a faith-based or spiritual practice;
> **Agreement**. When two or more people come together and agree with one another that something specific will be done;

Praise. Praise is an expression of love to God and of God;

Thanksgiving. Thanksgiving expresses thanks, gratitude, or appreciation for something;

Contemplation. Contemplation is a train of thought about something, such as scripture.

There are many types of meditations. This list is adapted from *headspace.com*:[POM10]

> **Focused (or breath) attention.** This form uses breath to focus attention, to anchor the mind and maintain awareness.
>
> **Body scan.** This technique is performed by a mental scan, from the top of the head to the end of your toes.
>
> **Noting.** This technique involves specifically noting what's distracting the mind. The thought is noted to restore awareness and then let go.
>
> **Visualization.** The meditator pictures something in their mind and then observes the mental and physical sensations.
>
> **Loving-kindness.** In this meditation, positive energy is directed to the meditator and then to others, which helps to let go of negative feelings.
>
> **Skillful compassion.** This form of meditation involves focusing on a person and paying attention to the sensations that arise.
>
> **Resting awareness.** This technique involves letting the mind rest. Thoughts may enter, but they are allowed to drift away.

Reflection. This technique asks a question and then becomes aware of the feelings that arise.

Zen meditation. This ancient Buddhist tradition involves following the breath, particularly the way it moves in and out of the body, and letting the mind just be.

Mantra meditation. This technique focuses on a mantra, a positive or loving syllable, word, or phrase.

Transcendental meditation. An instructor-led, fee-based, method of meditation.[POM11]

Yoga meditation. There are a variety of yogic meditations.

Vipassana meditation. Vipassana is an ancient Buddhist practice that allows the meditator to view the world in a new or different way.

Chakra meditation. Chakra meditation helps to cleanse and clear chakras and bring them back into balance.

Qigong meditation. "Qigong is a mind and body wellness practice integrating movement, posture, breathing, and awareness." [POM12]

Sound bath meditation. This meditation form uses bowls, gongs, and other musical instruments.

There are forms of prayer and meditation that combine two or more practices. The Catholic Rosary is one such form where prayers are counted using a string of beads. Buddhists also use prayer beads to count mantras or breaths during meditation.

Meditation and prayer are no longer confined to spiritual or devotional worlds. Mindfulness, a secular form of meditation,[POM13] has impacted business because of the positive benefits seen, including improved: focus, performance, efficiency, work/life balance, and communication.[POM14] As such, many companies offer mindfulness programs or resources such as meditation rooms.

Fred Grover Jr., MD, in his book *Spiritual Genomics*,[POM15] wrote a chapter called, "Shift Your DNA for Wellness and Longevity with Mindfulness and Meditation." In this chapter, Dr. Grover states, "In my opinion, the most important primary preventative strategy may be mindfulness – whether it prevents you from having heart disease or from hurting yourself or another in being over-stressed." From a scientific perspective, Dr. Grover cites a fascinating study on how meditation can increase telomere length.[POM16] Telomeres are protective end caps of DNA that shorten after cell divisions, and telomere shortening may be a powerful predictor of the lifespan of a species.[POM17]

Another interesting study showed that meditation improved brain size. Specifically, the regions associated with attention and sensory processing were more developed in meditators than in those who did not meditate.[POM18] The largest improvements were found in older participants.

I make daily meditation a priority. I meditate for about 15 to 20 minutes in the morning. When meditating by myself, I have enjoyed listening to Wayne Dyer's "I Am That I Am" meditation. Occasionally, I use a random meditation video from YouTube. Meditating with other people can be quite powerful. I have a meditation group that I usually meet and meditate with once per week. Do what works best for you.

My days, especially stressful days, are better when I meditate. Some of the ideas that I have written about in this book came to me while I was meditating.

Have Healthy Relationships

According to the National Institute of Health (NIH), strong social ties are associated with a longer life. In particular, healthy marriages are good for health. Married couples in healthy relationships "tend to live longer and have better heart health than unmarried couples." HHR1

We have many different types of human-to-human relationships. For example, we have family, friends, co-workers, neighbors, and intimate partners. Some of these relationships we choose and others we do not. Dr. Sheldon Cohen, a psychologist at Carnegie Mellon University, said that a diversity of relationships is important. In the NIH article, "Do Social Ties Affect Our Health?," Cohen said, "Involvement with other people across diverse situations clearly can have a very potent, very positive effect on health." HHR1

What makes our relationships healthy? There are many models of good, healthy relationships. Most of these models include characteristics such as trust, respect, intimacy, and vulnerability.

Conversations with God says, "The purpose of a relationship is to decide what part of yourself you'd like to see 'show up.'" CWG also suggests we often enter relationships for the wrong reasons. We are selfish if we enter relationships for what we can get out of them, rather than what we can contribute to them. Perhaps the most important relationship is with self. CWG says the following, "You must first see your Self as worthy before you can see another as worthy. You must first see your Self as blessed before you can see another as blessed.... If you cannot love yourself, you cannot love another.... You cannot give what you do not have."

How can we love ourselves without becoming selfish? In the article, "How To Love Yourself Without Guilt," HHR2 the author, Sandip Roy, says, "When you love yourself, it improves your relationships with others." He suggests that a way to love yourself is to "show acceptance, drop perfectionism, and act in self-compassion."

In 2015, I had a strong intuition that I had more growing to do. I acknowledge that I had been enormously selfish in all of my relationships up to that point in my life. I had been married for 17 years and we did not have children. I brought up the subject of divorce and my wife at the time readily agreed. Shortly after the divorce was finalized, and not by chance, I was invited to a self-improvement class. In one of the exercises, it became clear to me that I was weak not only spiritually but in my relationships as well. However, I was not sure what to do about it. What was important was that I had followed my intuition and opened the doors of possibility.

In a subsequent course, I realized how incredibly selfish I had been living my life. This particular day was the "high wire" day. I was feeling a bit cocky about this day because I had some experience with climbing and heights. That morning, the instructor said something I will never forget: "This is not Disneyland, and this is not a pull-up contest." A month earlier, I had won a pull-up contest in Las Vegas. The thought occurred to me that this experience was not about how many times I did the "rides" or how well I did them. A lot of people were intimidated by the exercises of this day and I realized that I could be there to support them. I know this may seem obvious to many people, but this was a novel concept for me. So, I decided to make that day about everyone but me.

Later that day, we were supposed to support the person behind us by giving them a hug and helping them out of their climbing gear after they finished the event. When the woman after me finished, I immediately started the process of helping her out of her gear. One of the coaches was observing and said, "Greg, give her a hug." Wow, I had forgotten I was there for emotional support. It was a great example that, if you want to break a bad habit or belief, the best way is to interrupt it while it is occurring. This exercise certainly did that for me.

After returning home from that class, I considered what I had learned. I am not sure where the idea came from –

we did over 40 different exercises that week – but I decided to call my father and tell him that I loved him. I had never heard him tell me this, and *I certainly had not told him that I loved him.* I was not sure what to expect. Because of his temperament, I never really knew "who" was going to show up when I called my father. Much to my surprise, after I told him, "I love you," he told me, "I love you too, and we need to do more of that."

An important factor in relationships and human longevity is sexuality. A study from England asked the question, "Sex and Death: Are They Related?" HHR3 In other words, is there a causal relationship between sexuality and longevity? In this study, the authors identified fewer orgasms being associated with earlier death. Many factors were considered in the study, including the possibility that sexual activity in older men could lead to instantaneous death. Indeed, even with these considerations, there was still a strong correlation with sexual activity and longevity in the studied men. I found a second, similar article related to sexuality and human longevity. This author questioned whether sexual activity was the causal factor of longevity or, rather, the relationship with another person that supported the longevity. The common factor seems to be relationships with other people.

Another wonderful relationship that we humans have that affects our health is our relationship with animals. Animals can serve as a source of comfort and support. Pets can positively influence the health of their owner. The study, "Pet Ownership and Cardiovascular Risk," published in the journal *Circulation*, highlighted several health benefits, including lower blood pressure and cholesterol, and better heart rate variability, an indicator of good heart health. Dog owners are more likely to get more physical activity compared with non-dog owners.[HHR4] This study concludes that there is substantial evidence that dog ownership, in particular, is associated with a reduction in risk factors for cardiovascular disease and better outcomes for those with established cardiovascular disease. Dr. Ann Berger from the NIH Clinical Center points out, "Dogs are very present. If someone is struggling with something, they know how to sit there and be loving. Their attention is focused on the person all the time." [HHR5]

Even caring for fish can have benefits. Diabetic teens caring for fish (feeding, checking water levels, and cleaning the tank) were more diligent about checking their glucose levels compared with teens without the same responsibility and, after three months of tending to their fish, their average glucose levels decreased.[HHR6]

Relationships are an ongoing evolution for me. My relationship with myself and with others has been changing and improving. The person I choose to be is joyful, present, accepting, and loving. This helps me relate to everyone better. My hope and expectation are that, if I get the chance to meet or interact with you, this is the person that shows up for you. I encourage you to decide who is going to show up in all of your relationships.

Angela Holloway is the angel who introduced me to CWG. I am so grateful for having her in my life. Besides introducing spirituality to me in a wonderful way, she has helped me and supported me in my personal growth. She has a son who has been a blessing to her and to me, especially since I do not have children. The best part is that we are learning, growing, and loving together. I love you, Angela. Thank you for being you.

Develop, nurture and be grateful for all of your relationships.

Be Purposeful and Service-Oriented

We all need reasons for living. Purpose and service-orientation are strong reasons for living. Regardless if that reason is "the plant," "the husband," or "the pet," any individual reason can stop being important. We need a reason or reasons that have endurance.

There are many cases – I am sure you can think of some yourself – after a person loses their purpose, they die soon after. I would like to share a personal example of this. In the 1990s, I worked as a systems manager in an automotive assembly plant. For many people, working in a manufacturing operation such as an automotive assembly plant brings much purpose and satisfaction. However, the expectations are relentless, and many people often have no life outside of the plant. The demands of the plant affected me physically as I started experiencing chronic headaches. Around 10:00 am, on the days I worked, I got headaches, and they were becoming more severe. Leaving the plant was, fortunately, an option for me, so I returned to a corporate office job. Not everyone has this option, and they grind through their jobs and their lives. Often these people turn to drugs and alcohol to help them cope with the stress of their situation.

About two years after I left the plant, I received a phone call from my former manager. "I thought you would want to know that 'Joe' has passed away." Joe was the assistant plant manager and a friend of mine. Joe went out of his way to be kind to me when I was at the plant, and I appreciated him. Joe retired about a year after I left the plant and lived less than a year after his retirement. I do not know what issues he had faced during his life, but I do know that, for Joe, the plant was his life. When his work at the plant was done, so was a significant reason for living.

Purposeful and service-oriented refers to both activities we get paid for and activities we do not get paid for. Most people need to work to pay their bills. This work is still service. It cannot be anything other than service to someone else. In some cases, the service is obvious. Healthcare workers see the service they provide to their patients. Factory workers also provide services that result in goods people use. If you think about it the other way around, everything that you have, including access to food, energy, and education, was brought to you through some form of service by other people. Our attitude about our work, knowing that it is of service to others, makes all the difference. Even if our work is not satisfying intrinsically, if that work supports a family or some other meaningful objective, it serves that important purpose.

Besides activities that provide payment, there are opportunities to be of service without expecting anything in return. This is often referred to as unconditional giving. In this sense, Samuel Johnson said, "The true measure of a man is how he treats someone who can do him absolutely no good." When we give unconditionally, I believe this is one of our highest acts of service.

Sadly, giving unconditionally was rare for me. For most of my life, my interactions with people, almost without exception, were transactions. This did not make them bad any more than this made them good, but the thought never occurred to me to do something for someone else without expecting something in return. I now realize how shallow my relationships were with almost everyone. I know that not having children contributed to this. I observe and am impressed with how generous my brother and sisters are with their children.

Lori Deschene, the founder of *Tiny Buddha, Simple Wisdom for Complex Lives*, wrote an article, "20 Ways to Give Without Expectations," where she provides a list of giving ideas.[PSO1] Similarly, Alexandra Franzen wrote, "50 ways to be ridiculously generous – and feel ridiculously good." [PSO2] Both articles are terrific, and I have selected several ideas from each to provide the following list:

Give money to someone who needs it and be anonymous about it.

Compliment strangers. Mention something highly-specific. "Way to rock that bow tie."

Let someone tell a story. Be present for them.

Ask someone at work, "What can I do to help you today?" Then follow through.

Become a member of a podcast you have been enjoying.

Send out an email designed to help somebody else. For example, make an introduction, send some encouragement, offer a helpful resource.

Apologize when you have acted selfishly. It sends the other person the message that they deserve to be treated with respect.

Listen to someone because you value their knowledge and appreciate their willingness to share it.

Tip someone generously. Decide what is a lot and then double it.

Buy a meal for a stranger.

Get excited about a small piece of good news, and say, "You did what? You are AMAZING!"

Assume the best intent from everyone, always.

What is your purpose? Do you need inspiration? I suggest cultivating interests and activities that bring you pleasure. Simple questions of "how can I help someone?" or "what do I love to do?" might provide clarity. Do you like to teach? Do you like to cook? Do you like to walk or hike?

If you are wondering what your service might be, in Thomas Frey's book, *Epiphany Z: Eight Radical Visions for Transforming Your Future*, Frey discusses and predicts the future of work.[PSO3] He paints an optimistic picture where humans are empowered to solve large-scale problems that have been impossible to solve before now. These problems and opportunities include:

Finding cures for diseases and aging;
Extending human abilities;
Correcting deviant human behavior;
Ending poverty;
Improving transportation;
Colonizing other planets;
Scientific and biological discovery; and
Mitigating the impact of natural disasters.

Perhaps one of these items challenges or inspires you. Still not sure about what your purpose could be? Take a look at your bucket list, or create a bucket list if you do not have one.

From whatever thoughts come, decide how you can be of service to someone else. It is never too late to do this. Do not be afraid to try. It is not only okay, but it is good to fail. Failing, in this context, means "I have identified something I do not like." Great. Move on to something else.

My friend, Larry, has donated over 70 gallons of blood, stem cells, and bone marrow.[PSO4] He started donating when he was 18 and was the youngest donor to reach the 70-gallon mark in Colorado. Larry is "addicted to saving lives." Back in 2000, his donated bone marrow helped extend the life of a woman for another year. His goal is to donate 100 gallons of blood. Larry, I thank you for your commitment to service.

I have volunteered at the Denver Rescue Mission and at the Food Bank of the Rockies. I appreciate the value of that service work, and in particular, I feel passionate about reducing poverty. I have an audacious goal that, by 2030, we, collectively, will raise and donate $25 million to provide food or services to people who need it. I have no idea how we will accomplish this goal. It does not matter. We get what we focus on, and this is what I choose to focus on.

The irony of life is that, when we focus on purpose and service to others, the Universe can brings us unimaginable prosperity, especially when this is not our objective. Of course, the ultimate irony is, when prosperity or fame happens, it is not important to us.

Are your beliefs holding you back? Some people do not believe that they are worthy of being happy or having meaningful work. If this is the case, addressing these underlying beliefs is critically important. Even if you do not believe, "I deserve meaningful work," you might believe, "My life is beginning to help me and other people."

Do not be afraid to express and be who you really are. Insist on it. It will add years, and perhaps more importantly, meaning to your life.

Be Happy and Present

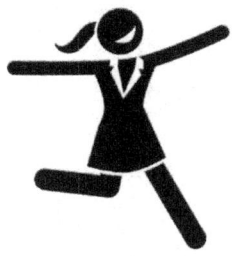

Research indicates that being happy can help us live longer. For example, a large study published in the journal, *Health Psychology*, found that happiness was significantly associated with lower risk of death in people with diabetes." [BHP1] The study noted that the effect was particularly powerful for those over 65 who reported higher levels of stress. Another study looked at 139 volunteers to determine how their positive emotional style (PES, their happiness) affected their ability to resist an illness after exposure to a virus. Increased happiness "was associated with lower risk of developing an upper respiratory infection." [BHP2] The authors of the study were excited about their results. In their conclusion they stated, "These results indicate that PES (happiness) may play a more important role in health than previously thought."

In 2009, Hilary Tindle, MD, and her colleagues studied the implications of optimism for over 97,000 women and how it affected their coronary heart health and mortality. This study confirmed several other studies showing optimism being associated with a "reduced incidence of coronary heart disease and total mortality." The authors suggested that the results of optimism directly affect our physiology, for example, our blood pressure, or indirectly through our behaviors, such as dealing with life's stressors in healthier ways.[BHP3]

A study published in August of 2019 investigated the survival of women from the Nurses' Health Study and men from the Veterans Affairs Normative Aging Study relative to how optimistic the subjects were. The study found that optimism, defined as the general expectation that good things will happen, is associated with an 11% to 15% longer lifespan, and a 50% to 70% greater likelihood of living to 85 or beyond. These results were determined to be independent of factors such as socioeconomic status, health conditions and behaviors (smoking or alcohol use), or depression.[BHP4]

Investigators have questioned why happiness or well-being would be associated with longevity. One finding was that senior adults who reported greater happiness tend to move their bodies more.[BHP4] Another finding is that happier people tend to eat better.[BHP5]

Understanding that happiness is not a function of the items around us is a valuable lesson I learned from traveling to over 30 countries. From these travels, I saw firsthand that some people are far less affluent than we are in the U.S. and yet, they are happy. A study from Purdue University found that, beyond a certain level of prosperity, after basic survival needs are met, more income does not lead to more happiness. People making more than about $100,000 per year tend to be less happy than those who make less, and happiness continues to decline with additional income.[BHP6] I believe that, with higher incomes, many people get caught up with their work and possessions and minimize their relationships and recreation.

Smiling is a powerful way to induce happiness in yourself and others around you. Smiling can "lift your mood, lower your stress, boost your immune system and possibly even prolong your life." [BHP7] According to Dr. Sivan Finkel, a cosmetic dentist at New York City's The Dental Parlour, "Even forcing a fake smile can legitimately reduce stress and lower your heart rate." I was having a conversation about smiling with my friend, Callen Borgias, an avid bicyclist and Colorado State Road Race Champion. He said, "When I'm really hurting on my bike, I sometimes remember to smile, and it actually results in a reduction in my perceived pain so I can go even harder. The key is remembering to do so."

For me, a path to happiness is being grateful. I have much to be grateful for and, sometimes, I just need to pause and think about it for a moment. I am grateful for freedom, prosperity, and the ability to live my dreams. I know this is possible because of the hard work and effort of many other people. I am grateful for the people who brought me food, the people who taught me, the people who made the thousands of parts that have gone into the cars I have driven, the people who have made the houses and apartments I have lived in, the people who brought me fuel for my car and electricity for my house, and on and on and on. When I think about my life this way, I remember that we are all one and are dependent upon one another.

"Our true home is in the here and the now. The past is already gone and the future is not yet here." Zen master, Thich Nhat Hanh.

All life is lived in the present moment. I am paraphrasing Eckhard Tolle when I say, past and future imaginings are nothing but illusions from the present moment. To me, this idea proposes a different paradigm of time – that we do not pass through time, but rather, time passes through us. I know this is contrary to our "experience," however, it seems that our essence does not change throughout our life. If we are fortunate enough, we experience ourselves as being born, as an infant, a child, a teenager, an adult, and an elderly adult until we die. We experience ourselves as single and in a relationship with someone else, as a leader and as a follower, as successful and as not successful. These aspects of our lives are all experiences that we have in the present moment. They never "happened" in the past or in the future.

We choose how we are being in every present moment. We choose to be happy or sad, friendly or mean, selfish or giving. We do not have to let circumstances determine how we are being. We can choose in advance.

Holocaust survivor Viktor Frankl decided to be cheerful, no matter what horrible circumstances he was facing.

When others asked him how he could be happy, he responded that he alone had control over his mind. He realized that a person could experience bliss by harboring the right thoughts.

Until recently, I almost always lived in the future. I became an expert at planning and even became a certified Project Management Professional. There is value in planning, but in my case, there was no balance between present and future. I would be exaggerating to say that I never lived in the present moment, but in my case, the present was typically forced on me rather than embraced by me. The future was always more enticing than the present moment. This was particularly true after I graduated from high school and started studying at the university in my hometown. I was highly motivated to get my engineering degree and move on from my hometown. As such, I did not have a typical college experience. My experience was mainly work and study with little time for fun or social activities.

I have become more present because of my spiritual awakening. I embraced the idea that "now" is all there is. Coming to this realization that there is nothing but the present moment provides many advantages. I am more aware of the beauty of everything around me and am not consumed with the burden of orchestrating a future, a future that may never come. I choose being present and happy. This is not automatic for me yet. I have to remind myself that, in every situation, there is something to be learned, experienced, or given to someone else.

This quote from Jack LaLane, one of the first fitness advocates, is perfect to drive these points home. "Life should be a happy adventure, and to be happy, you need to be healthy. Just take things one step at a time, and remember that everything you do takes energy to achieve. You need to plant the seeds and cultivate them well. Then you will reap the bountiful harvest of health and longevity!" BHP8

As simple as it sounds, the decision to be happy and present, can add years to our lives.

Use Aesthetics to Feel Better and Live Longer

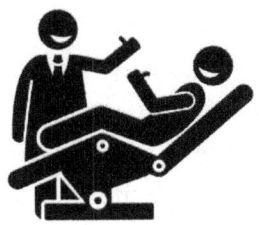

There are many aesthetic or cosmetic treatments available to help us look and feel better about ourselves.[AFB1] Aesthetic treatments are discretionary and impact our longevity indirectly because they can positively affect our self-image and behaviors. For this reason, I placed this topic in the spirit best practices.

Researchers have been investigating the connection between cosmetic procedures and improvements in self-esteem, social, and psychological feeling. Dr. Margraf and his colleagues investigated the outcomes from 808 people who either had or considered having a cosmetic procedure but did not. The group who had surgery was significantly happier with the specific physical outcome compared to the group who did not have surgery. More importantly, the group who had surgery scored significantly better than the group who did not on measures of "self-esteem, positive attitude, life satisfaction, and general feelings of attractiveness." [AFB2]

Beyond feeling good, researchers who studied women who had facelifts found that they lived ten years longer than those who did not.[AFB3] When asked why, Dr. Lyle Leipziger, chief of plastic surgery at North Shore University Hospital and Long Island Jewish Medical Center said, "I think that people who have plastic surgery are motivated, health-conscious individuals who are more likely to eat right, exercise, and take care of themselves. So it's not surprising that this type of person would have greater longevity."

Here is a list of aesthetic opportunities:

Grooming improvements
    Clothes
    Makeup
    Hair cut
    Hair color
    Nails
    Bathing/deodorant
    Shaving
Hair restoration or enhancement
    Head
    Eyelash
    Eyebrow
    Body hair removal
Skin enhancement
    Body skin
    Face
    Eyelid rejuvenation
    Lips
    Neck rejuvenation
    Hand rejuvenation

Teeth
  Straightening
  Whitening
  Implants
Body structure improvements
  Posture
  Vein reduction
  Nose (Rhinoplasty)
  Body sculpting
  Breast procedures
  Butt implants
  Calf augmentation

Of the many types of aesthetic options, some are simple and cheap while others are expensive. Clothing, hair color, posture braces, etc. can be low-cost, simple options. It is not necessary to wear clothes fashionable with people 30 years younger than you, but updating your clothes and grooming to age-appropriate current fashion can make you look and feel better and, at the same time, help you fit in with younger workers.

Surgical procedures carry risk and usually involve recovery time. In the U.S., plastic surgery is not covered by most health insurance plans. Because of this, this segment of healthcare acts as a competitive marketplace, meaning that it is possible to shop and price compare for different procedures.

There is an advantage to doing cosmetic treatments while you are younger so that the effects of aging are less pronounced. For example, BOTOX® relaxes the muscles of the forehead, thereby resulting in fewer wrinkles. Since these wrinkles tend to accumulate over time, the less time they are wrinkled, the less overall wrinkling occurs.

Skin is the largest and most visible organ of our bodies. Skin ages by wrinkling, hyperpigmentation, losing elasticity, and having a rough appearance.[AFB4] The major risk factors to our skin health include ultraviolet (UV) radiation exposure from sunlight,[AFB5] unhealthy eating, stress, lack of exercise, dehydration, smoking, obesity, and poor sleeping habits. Strategies to prevent damage and improve skin health include UV protection (clothing and sunscreens), hormone replacement, vitamin supplements, including vitamins C and D,[AFB6] linoleic acid, beta carotene, astaxanthin, coenzyme Q10, zinc, selenium, and compounds such as collagen and colostrum. Topical treatments include retinoids, water-soluble (glycolic acid) and lipid-soluble hydroxy acids (salicylic acid), ceramides, hyaluronic acid, and vitamins C and E.

I have had facial treatments including injectable BOTOX® and a Juvederm® facial injection. I have also used facial creams, including Retin A which requires a prescription. I am fortunate that I have most of the hair on my head and that it has only been slowly turning from blond to grey. Occasionally, I have colored my hair. During my bodybuilding experiences, I heard of some men opting for calf augmentation. I thought this was excessive.

It is possible to become obsessed with cosmetic procedures, spending hundreds of thousands of dollars on them. You are probably familiar with famous people who have fallen into this trap. The best practice is not to completely change your look, but to do enough to help you feel better about yourself. I saw a video describing one person's experience with cosmetic treatment and her attitude was, "Do what makes you happy, and do not care what others think." I support this.

Often, people use food as a reward for some goal or accomplishment, for example, getting ice cream after the ball game. Using food as a reward can have undesired consequences. A suggestion I offer is to purchase clothing or a cosmetic treatment as a reward for achieving a goal. For example, "After I lose 25 pounds, I am going to get a facial treatment." What you might want to consider is how you could provide one or more of these treatments for someone else in your life.

If you do not believe that you deserve any of the treatments mentioned, perhaps this is a good time to check and challenge your beliefs.

While you do not need to receive cosmetics treatments, you certainly are worthy of them.

Body-Based Longevity Best Practices

Have a Health Plan
Eat a Natural Diet
Consider Taking Basic Supplements
Move Your Body
Maintain Healthy Body Composition
Optimize Your Hormones
Avoid Toxic Substances

Have a Health Plan

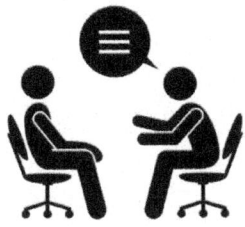

You alone are responsible for your health. Your health is not the responsibility of the government, your insurance company, your wife, husband, children, or even your doctor. However, the responsibility of your health care can be daunting because of the complexities of disease risk factors, medical and scientific terminology, insurance rules, and the costs and underlying economic incentives driving the healthcare system. Because of these complexities, it is valuable to form a team of health and medical providers that you can share your goals and unique circumstances with. With this team, you want to create a personalized healthcare plan.

Given that beliefs are critical to health, trusted relationships with our healthcare providers is essential. Short office visits make trusted relationships difficult for both patients and providers. Many doctors are opting out of traditional practice, opting for what has been coined "concierge medicine" providing personalized, specialized assessment, and prescriptive services. "My decision to convert my medical practice to concierge medical practice was based on my desire to be able to provide patients with the level of care I believe is essential to not only treat illness, but also to help them avoid becoming sick," says Jeffrey Friedman, MD, Director of Medicine at Community Health Associates.[HP1] Concierge doctors usually limit their practice to a small number of patients so that they can provide in-depth health care. Unfortunately, concierge doctors are not covered by traditional health insurance.

If you can afford a concierge doctor, that is a great option. Naturopathic doctors (NDs) are another possibility. Each state regulates the activities of NDs differently but, generally, they have the ability to offer natural treatments that do not involve drugs or surgery. In some cases, you can find both alternative and traditional providers within the same practice. In my case, I have seen traditional medical providers, a concierge doctor, and a naturopathic provider. I consider insurance doctors, dentists, chiropractors, massage therapists, and personal trainers part of my healthcare team.

Michael Fedewa, Jr., DO, from Duke University, recommends an annual physical exam to build trust with providers. Sangita Doshi, MD, agrees. In his article, "Your Annual Physical and Why It's Important," [HP2] he says, "Visiting your primary care provider for regular preventive care is one of the best ways to identify and treat health issues before they get worse." Dr. Doshi provides five reasons why an annual exam is a good idea.

Establishing a relationship with your doctor
Assessing your overall health

Updating your vaccinations
Screening for cancer and other diseases
Updating your medical records

Screenings can help find cancer and other diseases at an early stage before symptoms appear. When abnormalities are found early, they are usually easier to treat or cure. Depending on your situation, the overall health assessment may include screenings including[HP3, HP4]

Cholesterol
Blood glucose
Blood pressure
Body composition
Osteoporosis
Carotid artery plaque
Peripheral arterial disease
Cancer screenings, including breast, skin, colon, prostate, and lungs

The lab test results usually indicate when the results fall out of the normal range. These are talking points for you and your doctor.

Medical insurance in the United States is necessary because of the risk of medical bankruptcy due to unexpected medical procedures and treatments. Insurance is expensive and getting more expensive every year. I choose a high-deductible plan that is coupled with a health savings account (HSA). With an HSA, I can use pre-tax or employer-contributed money to select tests or certain preventative measures to benefit my overall health. This provides me with the most flexibility to determine what tests and treatments I would like to have performed. I often purchase tests in advance of seeing my doctor so we can discuss the results together.

Regardless of which insurance you have, *you do not have to let your insurer dictate your care*. This requires being active in your health care and understanding your prescriptions and treatments to get what *you* need and want, not necessarily just what the insurance company will pay for.

Your insurance may not cover blood screenings beyond cholesterol and glucose but, in most states, blood screens and other tests can be purchased yourself. Be as proactive as possible by purchasing what you can afford. Companies such as the Life Extension Foundation,[HP5] DirectLabs, and *Wellnessfx.com* provide tests you can pay for yourself. I have found that self-pay for these tests can be cheaper than after-insurance costs. In one case, I purchased a panel of tests through my doctor that I knew would cost around $200 from one of the online sources. In this case, I paid through my doctors' office and insurance. The tests cost $800 from the lab. My insurance company said that they negotiated a rate of $400 and that they would pay $200, resulting in me paying $200 for the tests. In other words, the insurance company passed the real cost of the test on to me.

Similarly, you might find that prescription savings programs like WellRx, GoodRx, or GoodRx Gold are cheaper options than your insurance co-pay. For example, I recently filled a 90-day supply of a prescription using GoodRx for $40. My insurance co-pay was $80. With GoodRx Gold, it would have cost me $20. GoodRx Gold comes with a monthly fee but could be a good choice depending on your needs. This is another example of how being active in your health care choices can result in savings and less hassle.

The point of disease prevention is to avoid or mitigate diseases and hospital visits as much as possible. Avoiding hospital visits also avoids the mistakes and complications that occur within the medical system. A rather somber analysis of the U.S. medical system, published in 2017, estimated that as many as 251,000 people a year in the U.S. die from medical errors.[HP6] While these numbers are disturbing enough, it is likely that the actual deaths are even higher, given that less than 10% of errors are thought to be reported. By contrast, about 635,000 people in the U.S. die every year from heart disease. If reported as a unique category, medical error would be the third-highest cause of death annually in the U.S.[HP7]

To get the best out of the medical system, I offer the following suggestions:

Be proactive;

Take responsibility for your health;

Build trust relationships with your healthcare team;

Share your health goals with clear and ongoing communication;

Create a health plan;

Do not let insurance dictate your care; and

Follow your health plan and modify it as needed to accomplish your goals.

No one cares about your health as much as you and you alone are responsible for your health. Be proactive and create a health plan for you.

Eat a Natural Diet

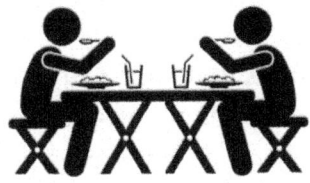

There are many benefits resulting from consuming a healthy, natural diet. Here are just a few:[END1]

Reduced cancer risk
Reduce cardiovascular disease
Stroke prevention
Healthier children
Strong bones and teeth
Weight control
Better mood
Improved memory
Better sleep
Better skin
Better sex[END2]

According to the best science, the evidence that we should eat unprocessed, whole foods, mostly plants, is undeniable. A 2014 comprehensive study from Yale University, "Can We Say What Diet Is Best for Health?" considered most of the common diets, including low carb, low fat, low glycemic, Mediterranean, paleo, vegan, and other diet plans. This meta-study concludes that the evidence supports "diets comprising preferentially minimally processed foods direct from nature and food made up of such ingredients, and diets comprising *mostly* plants." END3

I choose to eat foods that nature provides as much as possible. This type of diet is often referred to as a paleo or caveman diet because it attempts to emulate the foods our paleolithic ancestors consumed. I avoid processed and fried foods, such as sodas and French fries. I have difficulties digesting beans and lentils. Given this, when I have attempted a vegan diet, I have found it difficult to get an adequate amount of calories, protein, or to feel full. My solution is to eat some fish, free-range chicken, and eggs.

The Yale study does not suggest a 100% vegetarian or vegan diet. Proteins, actually the amino acids that construct protein molecules, are not optional; they are required for life. The daily Dietary Reference Intake of protein for sedentary people is 0.8 grams / kilogram of body weight.END4 For me, that is about 50 grams, but I am not sedentary. There is good research suggesting that older people, in particular, need protein in the amount of 1.0 to 1.2 grams / kilogram of body weight every day.END5 For me, that is 75 grams of protein. Since protein provides 4 calories per gram, 75 grams of protein equates to 300 calories. If I consume 75 grams of protein, comprised of meat, fish or eggs, this is approximately 15% of my total daily calories and is a low percentage consistent with the Yale study.

I appreciate that people who self-declare as vegan or vegetarian usually care about what they put in their bodies and tend to eat better than most people. The Yales study agrees that vegan diets, "when well constructed," are good for health. Some people, however, choose vegan or vegetarian diets in consideration of the environment or animal welfare and not necessarily for their health. I have observed some vegans and vegetarians eat a horrible diet of vegan junk food including pretzels, crackers, and fried potato chips. So, keep in mind, vegan does not necessarily mean unprocessed or healthy.

In his article titled, "Vegetarians live longer, but it's not because they do not eat meat," William MacAskill discussed the longevity of vegetarians.END6 He acknowledges that vegetarians live six to nine years longer than their non-vegetarian peers. The author questioned vegetarianism as being solely responsible for the longevity of vegetarians. He says vegetarians "are also more likely to exercise, be married, smoke less, and drink less alcohol – all factors that contribute to a longer life."

Two myths about food and eating are: 1) you cannot eat well when dining out, and 2) you cannot eat well while traveling domestically or internationally. You can usually make good choices wherever you are. In a restaurant, you are the boss. Even if the menu does not have what you want, ask for it. Ask for salads that have dressings on the side and for the cheese to be removed. Preparing in advance can help avoid situations with limited choices. I pack a meal or bring protein bars with me when I know my choices will be limited.

I can only think of a few times in my life that I have not been able to find something healthy to eat. One of those times was at a baseball stadium in California. The only food offered in the entire venue was through a hamburger chain. I was disappointed as I thought "everyone" in California wanted to eat well. I chose not to eat that night.

I was in Chengdu, China, for almost three weeks in 2012. Overall, the food quality in Chengdu was poor. Even though I found processed food and mystery meat everywhere there still were good choices. I stayed at a hotel where they had an international buffet for breakfast and dinner, and I found the local dish, "hot pot," to be a good choice. At the office, there was a food court with a sandwich shop. There were a couple of times when I had no idea what was being served and, once or twice, I decided it was better to fast than to eat.

Humans have a long-standing tradition of fasting, and fasting has been shown to extend lifespan.END7 Fasting for one or more consecutive days, or intermittent fasting practiced regularly, can provide powerful benefits. Intermittent fasting routines include fasting for 16 hours every day (the 16:8 method) and calorie restriction to around 500 calories for two days a week (the 5:2 method). Positive benefits from fasting include: assistance with weight loss, improved insulin resistance, decreases in various cardiac risk factors, including lower blood pressure, cholesterol, and triglyceride levels.

I have fasted, with supervision, for two, three, and five days. Fasting, in my case, meant I consumed only purified water. My fasts were good experiences. I was not hungry once my body adapted. In fact, I feel that fasting is easier than eating a small amount of food. Once I start the digestion process, by eating even a little, I find it difficult to stop eating. In addition, an all-day fast frees up several extra hours in the day from the time saved from preparing food, eating and cleaning up afterward.

I have mixed feelings about organic food production. In a perfect world, all of our food would be organic. Until relatively recently, *all food was organic*. However, there are some practical considerations. Organic methods are not as productive as conventional ones. If we have to burn down more rain forests to provide for organic farms, is that a good idea? I support sustainable and responsible farming. This is one way that we can all support each other.

It is especially important to listen to your body and, if you have questions about your situation, see a qualified professional. Registered dietitians and naturopathic doctors can be good sources of nutrition information. You can also explore websites including *diabetes.org*, *heart.org*, or *choosemyplate.gov* for more food and nutrition information. Many physicians acknowledge that they are not knowledgeable when it comes to food, nutrition, or exercise.[END8] The article, "Ignorance of Nutrition Is No Longer Defensible," [END9] supports this. My friend, Mark Chavez, MD, who wrote the book, *The 5 Habits of Healthy*

People: A Simple 5 Step Blueprint to Living a Long and Healthy Life, is a notable exception.

Make food good choices wherever you are.

Consider Taking Basic Supplements

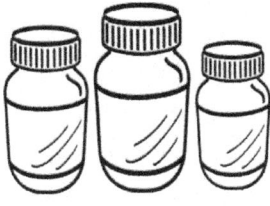

Since we do not eat as well as we should and the nutritional quality of much of our food has deteriorated,[SUP1] supplements can be helpful but are not a cure-all. Dr. Craig Hopp, from the National Institutes of Health (NIH), says, "There's little evidence that any supplement can *reverse* the course of any chronic disease." [SUP2] However, a 2005 study showed a complex dietary supplement extended lifespan and prevented or delayed some of the signs of aging in mice bred to experience accelerated aging.[SUP3] The NIH recognizes that supplements can *prevent* disease. The Dietary Supplement Health and Education Act of 1994 states, "The importance of nutrition and the benefits of dietary supplements to health promotion and disease prevention have been documented increasingly in scientific studies." [SUP4]

There are serious health consequences associated with vitamin and mineral deficiencies, especially for children and pregnant women. Even in affluent countries, many people are undernourished in one or more key nutrients while simultaneously consuming too many calories.[SUP5] Key reasons cited are copious consumption of processed foods and soils depleted of nutrients. If you need convincing, a study published in 2017 titled, "Risk of Deficiency in Multiple Concurrent Micronutrients in Children and Adults in the United States," investigated over 15,000 people aged 9 years and over found, "Thirty-one percent of the U.S. population was at risk of at least one vitamin deficiency or anemia." [SUP6] Another study advised, "Dietary supplements can be an important source of vitamins and minerals to prevent inadequate dietary intakes." Vegetarians and vegans, in particular, need to make sure they are getting enough vitamin B12, calcium, iron, and zinc.[SUP7]

In 2004, I read Michael Colgan, PhD's book, *Optimum Sports Nutrition*. I liked Dr. Colgan's content and writing style and attended several of his seminars. The first seminar I attended was an anti-aging seminar and discussed the benefits of exercise, food, supplements, as well as having a quiet mind (meditation) on longevity. An older gentleman asked me why I was interested in anti-aging. I told him that I wanted to preserve my vitality while I could because my belief was that this was easier than reversing aging. I went on to earn personal training certifications from the Colgan Institute and a certification as a Certified Sports Nutrition Advisor from the Cory Holly Institute.

Dr. Colgan and Cory Holly introduced me to the value of supplements, and I have been an avid consumer of supplements since I was diagnosed with low bone density in 2006. I take many of the supplements recommended by Somers' book *Bombshell*, but to take all of them would be quite expensive. I take the following supplements on a regular basis:

> **Whole Food Multivitamin.** I take a whole food multivitamin to "fill in the gaps" of my diet.[SUP8] Multivitamins are considered controversial because the evidence is, at times, weak that multivitamins prevent disease. There are several possible explanations, including that the doses taken are too low and the ingredients may be artificial or synthetic and, therefore, less bioavailable.
> **Vitamin D.** The benefits of vitamin D are many and include healthy bones, reduced risk of the flu, reduced risk of diabetes, and cancer prevention.[SUP9]
> **Fish oil.** There is evidence that fish oil can assist with heart health, skin health, and eye health.[SUP10]
> **Calcium.** I take calcium, magnesium, and related minerals to support bone health.[SUP11]
> **CoQ10.** CoQ10 helps in the production of energy in our cells' mitochondria. CoQ10 is also thought to help with diabetes and cancer prevention.[SUP12] Statin drugs can interfere with CoQ10 production.
> **Saw palmetto** is thought to help with men's prostate health. As an added bonus, it may help with urinary tract infections and prevent hair loss.[SUP13]
> **Chondroitin and glucosamine.** There is evidence to suggest that chondroitin and glucosamine are

anti-inflammatory and support healthy joints.[SUP14]

Trans-resveratrol. As mentioned earlier, resveratrol has been on the list of candidates considered as a possible calorie restriction mimetic. "Trans" indicates a specific chemical configuration of resveratrol. Resveratrol occurs in both trans and cis configurations. Trans is the active configuration and is what we want for maximum bioavailability.

NR, Nicotinamide Riboside. The Life Extension Foundation reports that resveratrol and NR are synergistic and are a powerful anti-aging duo that improve mitochondrial function and rejuvenate stem cells.[SUP15]

Acetyl-L-Carnitine. Research suggests that acetyl-L-carnitine can improve cognitive function and improve circulation.[SUP16]

CinSulin®, CinSulin® is a product containing purified cinnamon. Some, though not all studies, have shown that cinnamon can lower blood sugar.[SUP17]

As some vitamins and foods such as grapefruit can interact with medications, make sure to communicate with your healthcare team what you are currently or are considering taking. Get their guidance for what is best for you.

Pay attention to prescription instructions. After a medical treatment I had, I was given a course of antibiotics. I was supposed to take one dose in the morning and one in the evening for five days. On the last day, I read the instructions fully and they indicated that this medicine should not be taken with calcium. Calcium apparently deactivates the antibiotic which, of course, is not what I wanted to do.

Do your own research and talk with your healthcare providers to decide what supplements are best for you.

Move Your Body

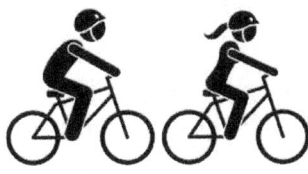

Movement is life. Our ancestors moved because they had to. In our modern world, moving our bodies is often not required and we have to consciously add movement to our routines. The most fundamental and practical movement is walking, and almost everyone can incorporate walking into their daily routine. Thom Rieck, of the Mayo Clinic, suggests a goal of walking 10,000 or more steps a day.[MYB1] A fitness tracker can help measure your steps, or you can time your walks to approximate your steps. Note: you should have proper medical clearance and monitoring before beginning any exercise program.

As in every other aspect of our lives, I am a firm believer in the concepts of belief and visualizations in exercise. In fact, our beliefs are the most important element of our exercise routine. If we do not believe we can climb the mountain or lift the weight, we will not. I start my workouts with a statement of gratitude (for our amazing body, for clean water, etc.) and an affirmation that "Every day I am getting stronger and stronger."

The physical activity guidelines provided by the U.S. Department of Health and Human Services are a well-regarded standard. The department provides a free, easy-to-read resource for physical activity called, "Physical Activity Guidelines for Americans." MYB2 The guidelines provide practical methods for children, adults, and older adults, to improve their health through physical activity. The key guidelines for adults are:

Move throughout the day. Any physical activity is better than none.

Perform aerobic activity of:
Between 2.5 hours and 5 hours a week of moderate intensity
Or
Between 1.25 hours and 2.5 hours a week of vigorous intensity
Or
An equivalent combination of moderate and vigorous-intensity activity.

Aerobic activity should be spread throughout the week.

Additional health benefits can be realized by engaging in more than 5 hours of activity a week.

Perform muscle-strengthening activities of at least moderate intensity that involve all major muscle groups 2 or more days a week.

The guidelines for older adults are the same as those for younger adults if no chronic conditions such as type 2 diabetes, cardiovascular disease, osteoarthritis, or cancer are present. The guidelines recommend gradual increases in activity for everyone. The National Academy of Sports Medicine (NASM) promotes the guidelines provided by the U.S. Department of Health and Human Services. I have held a NASM certified personal trainer certification for several years.

The many benefits [MYB3] from regular exercise include:

Increase your chances of living a longer high-quality life.

Strengthen your bones and muscles.

Help with weight control.

Improve your sexual health.

Reduce your risk of heart diseases and some cancers.

Help manage blood sugar and insulin.

Improve your sleep.

Improve your mental health and mood.

Reduce your risk of falls.

Help with smoking cessation.

I was a 120-pound weakling in high school and I did not compete in high school sports. After graduating from college, I moved to Florida and met a marathon runner who encouraged me to run with him, which I did. I was surprised by how good of a runner I was. Soon after I started running, I competed in my first running race. Once I started running and saw benefits from regular exercise, such as stress reduction, I emphasized fitness in my life. I went on to compete in many running races, and I won a half marathon in 2004.[MYB4] My running friend introduced me to a friend of his who was a bicyclist, and I started riding group rides along the coast of Palm Beach County, which was a lot of fun. I learned to swim and competed in several triathlons. In 2012, the year I turned 50, I committed to a year of triathlon training and racing. I hired a coach and competed in several races around the country. I was ranked in the top 8% of men in my age group according to the national triathlon ranking service.

In 2006 I was diagnosed with low bone density and I started weightlifting. While I was lifting in the company gym, a colleague asked me if I had ever considered bodybuilding and competing on stage. I wondered, was he talking to me? No, that thought had never crossed my mind, although the competitive aspect did appeal to me, and I decided to compete.

In amateur bodybuilding, there are two types of shows: natural shows that include drug testing and shows where there is no testing. I decided to compete in National Physique Committee (NPC) shows since I was prescribed testosterone to support my low bone density and I was not eligible to compete in natural shows. My first NPC bodybuilding show was in 2008. I competed in the bantamweight class, 143 pounds and below, and was the smallest man on stage. I did not let that deter me. I won the Colorado State bantamweight open division in both 2014 and 2015 at ages 51 and 52. I also took 3rd place in the 2015 Masters Nationals event in Pittsburgh for master's men 35 and over.[MYB5, MYB6] My last show was in 2016, where I competed against four men 30 years younger than me. I took 5th place, but I thought I looked great. I may compete again when I turn 60.

I will share with you some of my current physical fitness routines and recommendations. My current routine is six days a week of exercise, with each session lasting about an hour. I find that a mix of three days of weightlifting and three days of cardiovascular exercise works well for me.

I bike, hike, and use an elliptical rowing machine for cardiovascular activities. During my triathlon season in 2012, I developed a hip problem that has limited my running. To substitute for running, I have been hiking. The last two summers, I hiked 17 different 14,000-foot mountains in Colorado.

I prefer one light-, one moderate-, and one high-intensity cardio workout per week. The company, Polar, which manufactures heart rate tracking devices, defines heart rate zones as:[MYB7]

Polar Cardio Heart Rate Zones

Intensity	% of Maximum Heart Rate
Very Light	50% to 60%
Light	60% to 70%
Moderate	70% to 80%
High	80% to 90%
Maximum	90% to 100%

Maximum heart rate is often estimated at 220 minus your age. For example, I am 57, so my maximum theoretical heart rate is 163 beats per minute. 60% of 163 beats per minute is 98 beats per minute. At least occasionally, I like to train with a heart rate monitor so that I know that I am close to my target zones and can feel what a 60% or an 80% effort is like.

When lifting weights, I only stress one body area each week. For example, one day a week is leg day and another day is back, arms, and abs. Rest is very important. We do not get stronger during our run or while in the gym. The body overcompensates and grows stronger after the stress of exercise is removed.

There are many opinions and myths related to exercise and I will discuss a few. First, there is no perfect exercise. My suggestion is to do whatever you enjoy doing. Second, if there were a perfect exercise, it would only be perfect for a few weeks or months at most. Our bodies adapt quickly and, we should change our exercise and movement patterns to provide new challenges for our bodies. Third, especially in the absence of a sensible diet, it is impossible to exercise your way to weight loss. About the only people I have seen who are thin because of exercising are competitive runners and triathletes. Remember this saying: abs are made in the kitchen.

If you do decide to exercise, do it right. What matters to our bodies is the stress we place on the muscle, not how much weight we lift. There are many ways to cheat when lifting weights. Swinging hips and arms introduces momentum that allows much larger weights to move on their own. This is not recommended or beneficial. The body responds to resistance exercise that emphasizes good form and that maximizes muscular contraction known as "time under tension."

Three sets of eight repetitions of an exercise is considered standard, but this should be varied over time. NASM recommends a repetition (rep) cadence of two seconds of concentric contraction and two seconds of eccentric contraction.[MYB8] That means each rep is four seconds and a set of eight reps takes 32 seconds. Most people finish a set much faster than this.

If you do not know what to do or where to start, engage a coach or trainer. A certified personal trainer can assess your current fitness, create an exercise plan tailored to your needs and assist you in implementing and following the plan safely and effectively. Having someone observe and make sure your posture and form are good is not only helpful but much safer for long-term health. Eventually, you will be able to train yourself so that you will not have to depend on a trainer.

I have used trainers and coaches for both weightlifting and triathlon racing. Trainers and coaches always introduce me to new ideas and push me harder than if I were training by myself.

Two other aspects of physical health that I work on are flexibility and agility. Particularly as we age, both flexibility and agility exercises are essential to include in order to avoid and mitigate falls that can result in debilitating bone fractures. Both agility and flexibility can be improved at any age. A qualified trainer can assist you with ways to improve both.

If you are not moving your body as much as you want to, set a goal for yourself. Specific, measurable, attainable, realistic, and time-measured (SMART) goal-setting works particularly well with weight training and endurance exercise.

Here is an example of a SMART goal. Sarah monitored her walking for a few days and realized she was only walking about 5,000 steps a day. She wants to do more, but she is not sure how quickly she can ramp up. Her SMART goal is: "Walk 10,000 or more steps five days a week within eight weeks." The goal is SMART because it is:

Specific. It is clear what Sarah's goal is.

Measurable. A fitness tracker can automatically measure Sarah's steps and provide her reports of her activity.

Attainable. Based on her current fitness level, Sarah can increase her walking 10% per week and safely achieve the goal.

Realistic. Sarah's goal is realistic because she has assessed her current condition and can gradually increase her activity to meet the goal.

Time-Measured. The goal is time-bound to eight weeks.

Once Sarah has achieved this goal, it is important for her to set a new SMART goal to maintain her achievement. A second goal would be to continue walking 10,000 or more steps five days a week for at least eight weeks to form a lifelong habit.

Do what you enjoy and what you can manage in your daily routine. You can incorporate additional movement into your daily activities by walking more, taking the stairs, gardening, dancing, or golfing.

Some exercise or movement is better than none. Strive for progress not perfection.

Maintain Healthy Body Composition

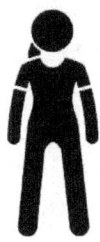

Body composition is defined as the proportion of body fat to total weight. There are many adverse health outcomes related to poor body composition. For example, a 2012 study found that people with a poor body mass index (BMI) had a weakened immune system.[HBC1] Being overweight can trigger immune reactions in the brain that disrupt memory and thinking.[HBC2] A 1999 study estimated that 280,000 people died in the U.S. every year as a result of obesity.[HBC3] The situation has only gotten worse in the last 20 years. In the 2015-2016 survey, 18.5% of children and nearly 40% of adults were obese.[HBC4] These were the highest rates ever documented by the National Health and Nutrition Examination Survey.

If you are moving your body regularly and eating a largely plant-based diet, you likely have a healthy body composition. In nature, it is unusual to see overweight animals. Humans who have to hunt and farm their own food generally are not overweight because so much effort is necessary to obtain food. This was true in the Biosphere II experiment, where the participants were slowly starving because they could not grow enough food to survive in the enclosed space. In the modern world, food can be obtained with little physical effort and people do not realize how much they eat and how little physical activity they perform.

How is body composition determined? The challenge is that there is no method, other than dissection, that can measure body fat exactly. So, every method for determining body composition is an estimate. There are several methods available for estimating body composition and they all have advantages and disadvantages.

The simplest body composition estimate is BMI. BMI is an indicator of body composition based on height and weight. It was developed in the 1830s by a statistician from Belgium.[HBC5] The calculation is simply a person's weight (in kilograms) divided by their height (in meters) squared.[HBC6]

I will manually calculate my BMI based on my measurements. I weigh 140 pounds. 140 pounds is 63.6 kilograms. I am 65 inches tall. 65 inches is 1.65 meters. So, my BMI is 63.63 kilograms / (1.65 meters x 1.65 meters) which produces a BMI of 23.4. As the BMI chart indicates, my BMI is in the healthy range.

There are many online calculators that you can use to calculate your BMI. Knowing your BMI, the following guidelines are available to assess your body composition.[HBC7]

BMI Ranges and Body Composition Status

BMI Range	Body Composition Status
Below 18.5	Underweight
18.5 – 24.9	Normal or Healthy Weight
25.0 – 29.9	Overweight
30.0 and Above	Obese

BMI has its critics and does not measure everyone correctly, especially heavyweight bodybuilders who have a disproportionate amount of muscle relative to their height.

Other methods for estimating body composition include:[HBC8]

> **Skinfold measurements** can be performed by a qualified personal trainer.
> **Electrical impedance** measurements are found in some electronic scales.
> **DEXA scan equipment** can be found in diagnostic centers and some doctor's offices.
> **Hydrostatic weighing** requires specialized equipment that is not commonly available.

From any of these methods, a body fat percentage calculation is accurate within a couple of percentage points.

The results from different body fat measurement methods can vary slightly. As an example, within two weeks, I was measured at 8% body fat using a skinfold calculation, 10% on an electronic scale, and 12% from a DEXA scan. These results could be interpreted as if I gained body fat, when, in actuality, I had not. Use only one measurement method to monitor your body composition trend. If body fat measurements from your electronic scale, week over week, are 25%, 22%, 23%, 20% and then 19%, you know that you are trending lower.

Healthy body fat levels are different for adult men and women. The American Council on Exercise (ACE) offers the following guidelines:[HBC9]

ACE General Body Fat Percentage Categories

	Women (% fat)	Men (% fat)
Essential Fat	10-13%	2-5%
Athletes	14-20%	6-13%
Fitness	21-24%	14-17%
Average	25-31%	18-24%
Obese	32% +	25% +

If a 45-year-old man has a BMI of 30 and is measured at 34% body fat by DEXA and 30% by electrical impedance, then he can know that he has a poor body composition and should discuss this situation with his doctor.

When I was bodybuilding and posing on stage, I was in the 5.5% to 6.5% body fat range. Professional male bodybuilders temporarily drop to the 3% to 4% range for their shows. This low percentage of body fat is quite unnatural and can be dangerous. For bodybuilders, very low body fat is artificial and temporary.

If your body composition is not where you want it to be, work with your healthcare team to create a SMART goal and a plan that you can use to achieve your target weight.

You deserve health and vitality and can achieve anything you set your mind to.

Optimize Your Hormones

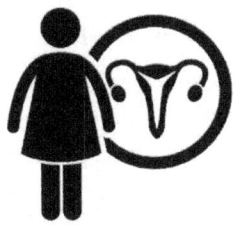

The endocrine system is a set of organs and glands that produces and secretes hormones that are transported in fluids such as blood or lymph to stimulate specific cells or tissues to regulate metabolism, growth, reproduction, and response to stress, among other functions.[OYH1] As such, this system has "a major influence on aging and longevity."[OYH2] In typical human aging, the pituitary-based hormones, including the hormones of the adrenals, ovaries, and testes, decline after peaking during our 20s or 30s.[OYH3]

The role of sex hormones in men and women is different. For example, the implications of low testosterone in men are:[OYH4]

> Loss of sex drive
> Lower sperm production
> Lower muscle mass and strength
> Fat distribution changes
> Lower bone density
> Lower red blood cell production

There has been controversy whether hormone replacement therapy causes prostate cancer. The 2016 meta-analysis of 26 trials concluded this was not the case. "Prostate cancer appears to be unrelated to endogenous testosterone levels." [OYH5] In some circumstances, hormone therapy can be an adjunct in treating cancers.[OYH6] This is great news for men, including myself as I will be on testosterone replacement therapy for the rest of my life. All the men I have talked to who have been prescribed testosterone replacement therapy say it is the best thing that ever happened to them and they are not interested in stopping the therapy.

For women, the situation is complex. The main sex hormones that are involved in women's health are estrogen, progesterone, and testosterone. The effects on women due to menopause is the reduction of estrogen and progesterone and can cause:[OYH7]

Hot flashes
Fluctuating moods
Weight gain
Painful sex/vaginal dryness
Insomnia
Lower bone density

Two terms related to hormones are bioidentical hormones and compounding. Bioidentical hormones are those that are molecularly identical to hormones produced by humans. According to the FDA, "compounding is a process of combining, mixing, or altering ingredients to create a medication tailored to the needs of an individual patient." [OYH8]

In 2002, the Women's Health Initiative study recommended stopping their trial related to administration of estrogen plus progestin (a non-bioidentical form of progesterone) because breast cancer incidents in the trial exceeded safety protocols.[OYH9] Controversy exists related to the outcome of this study. It has been proposed that, if bioidentical hormones had been used instead of synthetic, the results might have been much more positive.[OYH10]

In 2006, I was volunteering for my neighbor, who was leading the bone health division of the American College of Sports Medicine. Her lab was testing the bone health of cyclists and was discovering that the bone health of many cyclists was poor. The technician I was working with asked me if I wanted my bone density measured via a DEXA scan and I agreed. I was diagnosed with osteopenia, low bone density. This diagnosis was both surprising and fortunate since it was discovered while I was relatively young.

Osteopenia and the more severe osteoporosis are serious health issues and often not diagnosed until a person falls and breaks a bone. If the fracture is a hip, the repercussions can be fatal. A 2010 study titled, "Excess mortality in men compared with women following a hip fracture," found that 37.1% of men with hip fractures died within 12 months.[OYH11]

The technician suggested that I consult with my doctor about strategies for addressing this issue. My doctor ran blood work on me and discovered that my testosterone was low. He said, "We have found the smoking gun." Since steroids are anabolic, which means tissue building, I was prescribed testosterone. There are many testosterone supplementation options available for men, including gels, compounded creams, and injectables. I self-inject testosterone cypionate once per week. I also take anastrozole to limit the conversion of testosterone to estrogen. Too much estrogen in men can cause problems.[OYH12]

In addition to supplementing with testosterone, I started taking supplements that support bone health and I began weightlifting. Both weightlifting and gymnastics are known to improve bone density. I responded quite well to the therapy. The University of Colorado Health Sciences department published a short paper describing my results.[OYH13] Interestingly, in 2012, I limited my weightlifting to focus on triathlon training. At the end of my triathlon season, I had another DEXA scan and my bone density had decreased significantly. Since then, I have balanced cardiovascular exercise and weight training, and my bone density has stabilized.

Hormone levels can be assessed from a blood sample. Typical insurance plans generally do not cover hormone testing unless you have a specific situation like mine. However, in most states, you can order hormone blood tests and self-pay.

Hormone replacement and balancing may be just what you need. Talk with your healthcare team about the potential benefits and risks for your situation.

Be proactive. Get your hormone levels tested and consult with your doctor. Then take action, if needed.

Avoid Toxic Substances

This best practice recommendation is to avoid toxic substances in the food we eat, in the fluids we drink, in the air we breathe, and in anything that touches our skin.

If you do an internet search for toxic substances, you may conclude that everything is toxic. Actually, almost everything is toxic at some dose, quantity, or exposure level. Water is a good example. Obviously, too little water is a problem, but too much water in the body can lead to a condition called hyponatremia, which means low sodium concentration. This situation disrupts many normal cellular processes and can lead to death.

According to the Life Extension Foundation, detoxification is the process of removing unwanted fat-soluble compounds from the body.[ATS1] The liver and other organs convert the toxin into an inert, water-soluble form that is subsequently excreted. The Life Extension Foundation article says, "Given the sheer number of diverse enzymes and transport proteins involved in metabolic detoxification and its related pathways, it is no surprise that detoxification depends on, and is sensitive to, a large number of dietary factors." The message is that a good diet helps with both avoiding toxic substances and providing the body with the necessary nutrients to facilitate detoxification.

Here are a few toxic substances found in food or the environment that we should be aware of and manage our exposure to.[ATS2]

Cigarette Smoke. One toxic substance that should not surprise anyone is smoke from cigarettes. According to the American Cancer Society, "Tobacco smoke is made up of thousands of chemicals, including at least 70 known to cause cancer." [ATS3] Some of the carcinogens, agents known to be capable of producing cancer, found in tobacco smoke include:

> Hydrogen cyanide
> Formaldehyde
> Lead
> Arsenic
> Radioactive elements, such as uranium
> Benzene
> Carbon monoxide
> Polycyclic aromatic hydrocarbons

Vaping or e-cigarettes have become popular recently. While vaping may expose the user to fewer toxins, vaping is still bad for the user's health and, possibly, anyone within close proximity to the exhaled aerosol particles.[ATS4]

There are many treatment programs and resources available that can help anyone who wants to stop smoking.

Refined Sugar. What is being referred to here is sugar that is processed and refined, and then added to food, not sugar that naturally occurs in whole fruits and vegetables. There are many reasons to avoid refined sugar[ATS5, ATS6] because refined sugar:

Accelerates aging

Increases the risk of obesity, diabetes, and heart disease

Causes tooth decay

Can cause gum disease

Can suppress immune function

Negatively affects the brains of children and adults

Increases stress levels

Negatively affects mood

Fructose is a special type of sugar that is found in some whole fruits and vegetables. Manufacturers often sweeten their products with high fructose corn syrup because it is inexpensive. Until recently, humans were never exposed to high concentrations of fructose. At higher concentrations, fructose has been associated with insulin resistance, increasing bad cholesterol, and leptin resistance, which could contribute to obesity.[ATS7]

The American Heart Association recommends that men limit their sugar intake to 150 calories or 37.5 grams per day. Women should limit their sugar to 100 calories or 25 grams per day.[ATS8] This is a low limit. A single can of soda may contain more than 30 grams of sugar.

With ubiquitous availability of processed foods, adhering to the recommended amounts of sugar is challenging. The best way to know how much sugar we are consuming is to monitor food consumption with a food diary. There are many tools available to assist with this.

Avoid processed foods with added sugar. Keep in mind that fruit juice is highly processed and contains high concentrations of sugar. Check the labels.

Sodium. Just like water, there is the right amount of sodium (salt) in our diets. For most people, eating a diet low in processed foods will provide the proper amount of sodium. Hyponatremia (low sodium in the body) is rare. The United States Department of Agriculture recommends a daily sodium intake of less than 2,300 milligrams (2.3 grams).[ATS9]

Refined Vegetable Oils, Seed Oils, and Trans Fats. These oils are processed and tend to cause health problems. From an evolutionary perspective, humans never consumed concentrated seed oils such as soybean oil. The challenge with many refined oils is that they contain an unusually high level of omega-6 fatty acids. Our bodies are expecting a certain ratio of omega-6 to omega-3 oils. Too much omega-6 oils can lead to blood clots and strokes. Further, processing oils changes the chemical bonds within the molecule from the natural "cis" configuration to "trans." According to the American Heart Association, trans fats increase the risk of developing heart disease, stroke, and type 2 diabetes.[ATS10]

The obvious recommendation is to use processed oils sparingly, with olive and avocado oils being the best choices. Fats from most nuts, such as walnuts, and seeds, such as flax or pumpkin, and avocados are generally considered healthy.

BPA Bisphenol-A (BPA) is a chemical found in plastic containers of many common foods and beverages. The effect of this chemical on humans and animals has been studied extensively. Many studies show harmful health effects attributable to BPA. However, studies supported by the chemical industry and the FDA state that the levels most humans are exposed to are safe.[ATS11] There is evidence that BPA is removed from our bodies fairly quickly, but there may be a long latency between exposure and consequences which makes it difficult to determine if BPA is responsible for causing problems.[ATS12]

Who can we believe and what should we do? To stay on the safe side, you can avoid the BPA from foods in cans or bottles by eating a minimally processed diet. Choosing BPA-free containers and avoiding food microwaved in plastic containers are also good ideas.

Mercury. Mercury causes direct damage to cells and their functions.[ATS13] Entire organ systems can be affected. Further, mercury accumulates in animals over time. Tony Robbins thought he was making a healthy choice by consuming large amounts of tuna and swordfish.[ATS14] These two fish are long-lived and tend to have high levels of mercury. Robbins was suffering from fatigue and memory problems. When he was checked, Robbins' mercury blood levels were measured at a life-threatening level. Fortunately, he was able to obtain treatment that rapidly lowered his mercury level.

I learned from Robbins' mistake. I limit my consumption of tuna and swordfish to a few times a year. I do enjoy salmon weekly. Salmon is a short-lived fish that does not accumulate as much mercury as tuna. I also buy fish oil that has been molecularly distilled to remove toxic substances, including mercury.

Lead and other heavy metals. The toxic results from lead exposure have been widely reported in the U.S. and Canada, and lead exposure is generally controlled in these countries. However, lead control in developing countries should not be taken for granted. Be cautious about products, especially children's products, from developing countries.[ATS15] This is easier said than done because global sourcing makes it difficult to understand the origin of products and their components.

Alcohol. The World Health Organization's International Agency for Research on Cancer categorizes alcohol as "carcinogenic to humans." [ATS16] The World Health

Organization estimates that 4% of all deaths worldwide are attributable to alcohol, and alcohol is the leading risk factor for mortality among males aged 15-59.[ATS17]

After I graduated from college, I moved to Florida and I started drinking regularly. Fortunately for me, I also started running and cycling. It was clear to me that I could not run or bike ride as well the morning after drinking. One Friday after work, I had a few drinks during happy hour. Afterwards, I was driving aggressively through traffic, but a voice in my head suggested that I slow down. I immediately reduced my speed to the legal limit and looked over my right shoulder to see a state trooper staring at me. I was fortunate that I was not pulled over, as I was probably over the legal blood alcohol limit. I realized that I needed to change my consumption of and attitude toward alcohol. I decided to minimize consumption of alcohol and focused on physical fitness.

If you have problems with alcohol or any addictive substance, get help and treatment. Support groups can be a powerful source of recovery and community.

One final thought on avoiding toxic substances is cinnamon. I had been taking low-cost cinnamon supplements as part of a non-pharmaceutical strategy for managing my blood glucose. Some studies have shown cinnamon to be beneficial in managing blood glucose levels, but cinnamon often contains a compound called coumarin that can be toxic to the liver.[ATS18] As a result of my research on toxic substances for this book, I decided to purchase a cinnamon supplement, CinSulin®, that has been purified to remove coumarin. This is a good example of why it is important to purchase products from trusted sources with reputations for good quality control.

Mind-Based Longevity Best Practices

Protect Your Brain
Choose the Right Amount of Stress
Sleep Seven Hours Per Night

Protect Your Brain

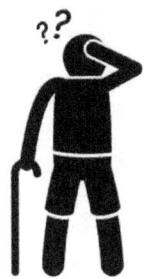

Unfortunately, aging adults are increasingly susceptible to neurodegenerative diseases, including Alzheimer's, Parkinson's, and Lou Gehrig's disease. 37% of people over age 85 are suspected of having Alzheimer's dementia.[PYB1] Currently, there is no cure for Alzheimer's and slightly over 4% of deaths per year are attributable to Alzheimer's.[PYB2]

Alzheimer's disease is a chronic condition with symptoms developing gradually. The Alzheimer's Association provides this list of signs of Alzheimer's or other dementias.

Memory loss that disrupts daily life

Challenges in planning or solving problems

Difficulty completing familiar tasks at home, at work, or at leisure

Confusion with time or place

Trouble understanding visual images and spatial relationships

New problems with words in speaking or writing

Misplacing things and losing the ability to retrace steps

Decreased or poor judgment

Withdrawal from work or social activities

Changes in mood and personality

Significant research is focused on investigating causes and finding cures for Alzheimer's disease. Lines of research include drugs, hormones, light, sound, and electronic stimulation.[PYB3] The Alzheimer's Association says Alzheimer's is "not a normal part of aging" and offers the following practices to reduce the risk of getting Alzheimer's and other dementias:

Manage cardiovascular risk factors (especially diabetes, obesity, smoking, and hypertension).

Engage in regular physical activity.

Eat a healthy diet.

Engage in lifelong learning.

Have a mentally stimulating job.

Engage in mentally stimulating activities.

Remain socially active.

Similarly, the Kaiser Permanente Washington Health Institute offers several suggestions to protect your brain.[PYB4]

Control cardiovascular risks.
Exercise three or more times per week. People who exercise three or more times per week have a significantly lower risk of developing dementia
Avoid a high sugar diet. Research has shown that high blood sugar raises the risk of developing Alzheimer's disease and dementia.
Do not smoke. Smoking is associated with faster cognitive decline.[PYB5]
Avoid overmedication. Overmedicating can subject people to dangerous drug interactions. Certain medications are linked to a slightly higher risk of dementia.
Avoid or moderate alcohol consumption. Avoiding alcohol is especially important when taking certain medications. For men, moderate drinking is defined as two drinks per day. For women, one drink per day is considered moderate drinking.
Limit stress. Older brains have a more difficult time coping with the stress hormone cortisol.
Get adequate sleep. Inadequate sleep is associated with slower thinking and the development of dementia

Avoid head injury. Take necessary precautions to avoid accidents and falls.

Physical activity does not need to be intense or strenuous to be beneficial for our brains. A study in Germany looked at the effects of dancing in older subjects. The study authors observed that dancing seems promising for improving both balance and brain structure. Dancing is considered good therapy because it combines aerobics, sensory, motor, and cognitive skills with a low risk of injury.[PYB6]

The other physical activity that appears to be especially beneficial to the brain is walking in nature. In one study, a 90-minute walk in a natural setting decreased focus on negative thoughts. The nature walk also reduced neural activity in an area of the brain linked to mental illness. The same 90-minute walk in an urban setting did not offer the same benefits.[PYB7]

A meta-analysis examining the effects of dietary interventions on symptoms of depression and anxiety determined that diet "plays a role in the treatment and self-management of depressive symptoms across the population." [PYB8] Mushrooms, in particular, could be helpful to stave off cognitive impairment. The National University of Singapore studied seniors and found that those who eat more than two standard portions of mushrooms, defined as three-quarters of a cup of cooked mushrooms, per week may be 50% less likely to suffer mild cognitive impairment.[PYB9]

Several substances have been associated with improved brain function. These include fish oil, resveratrol, and caffeine.[PYB10] The effects on brain health of the components of fish oil, DHA and EPA, have been studied extensively. Both separately and in combination, DHA and EPA are associated with improved memory, reaction times, and mood.[PYB11, PYB12]

Eight weeks of meditation measurably improved people's brains in one study. The researchers noticed improvements in several regions of the brain. The brains of the new meditators saw a reduction of the amygdala, which is associated with fear, anxiety, and aggression. The size reduction correlated to reduced stress levels in the study participants.[PYB13, PYB14]

Meditation moves the brain from the more active beta state, 15 to 45 Hz, to the calmer theta state, 5 to 8 Hz. Sleep produces even calmer brain states of 1.5 to 4 Hz.[PYB15] We know that muscles need time to recover from the stress of exercise. Therefore, it stands to reason that the brain, like muscle, requires both stimulus as well as recovery for good health. I propose that the theta state induced by meditation could provide a type of recovery that is not possible from the delta state produced by sleep.

Lumosity™ has developed games and exercises to protect and improve your brain in as few as 3 minutes per day.[PYB16]

Protect your brain by living the spiritual and body best practices, and adding brain stimulating activities, dancing, and walks in nature.

Choose the Right Amount of Stress

I heard Tony Robbins say that there is a healthy amount of stress. Too little stress or stimulation and we are bored. Too much stress and we go crazy and can fall apart. The following quote from the study, "The impact of stress on body function: A review," supports this idea: "It is believed that mild stress facilitates an improvement in cognitive function, especially in the case of virtual or verbal memory. However, if the intensity of stress passes beyond a predetermined threshold, which is different in each individual, it causes cognitive disorders, especially in memory and judgment." STR1

Stress affects our brain in at least two ways, our memory and our ability to learn. The hippocampus is responsible for the processing and storage of short-term memory as well as cognition. Research indicates that stress can result in atrophy, neurogenesis disorders, and reduction in the volume of the hippocampus portion of the brain. Stress was shown to decrease the number of dendritic branches, the number of neurons and for "structural changes in synaptic terminals." STR1

It is well known that stress affects more than the brain. Stress affects the immune system, the cardiovascular system, the gastrointestinal (digestive), and the endocrine system.[STR1]

What is stress? "Stress is the body's reaction to any change that requires an adjustment or response. The body reacts to these changes with physical, mental, and emotional responses." Based on research from endocrinologist Dr. Hans Selye, the three stages of stress are:[STR2]

> **Alarm.** A fight or flight response that releases stress hormones adrenaline and cortisol and raises blood pressure.
> **Resistance.** The body can recover if the stress is relieved. If the stress is not relieved, the body continues to excrete stress hormones and blood pressure remains elevated.
> **Exhaustion.** The result of prolonged unresolved stress resulting in fatigue, burnout, and depression.

Our modern lifestyles produce chronic stresses that are not normal from an evolutionary perspective. If we do not deal with stress appropriately, "stress can kill you," said Dr. Diana Gall in an article published in *The American Institute of Stress*.[STR3]

What are some ways of coping with too much stress? The obvious and best approach is to avoid chronically stressful situations. For example, when I was working in the auto assembly plant, I developed canker sores on the cheeks of my mouth. I realized that these sores were related to stress because I remembered that I would get them during final exam week when I was in school. For me, the plant was a stressful situation and I did not have good coping mechanisms. Ultimately, my way to manage that stress was to leave the plant.

For those who have chronically stressful jobs, such as first responders and air traffic controllers, it is important to lower the effects of stress. Here is a list of stress reduction techniques:STR4, STR5, STR6, STR7

Exercise
Pray or meditate
Take a walk
Get or give a hug
Aromatherapy
Be creative artistically
Eat better
Enjoy your favorite leisure activity
Yoga
Express gratitude for what you have
Accept what is
Reassess your priorities
Get social support
Massage
Tai chi
Biofeedback
Reduce or eliminate stimulants like caffeine
Journal
Chew gum
Laugh
Spend time with family

Learn to say No
Spend time with your pet
Let go of perfectionism

There are certainly times when professional help is appropriate and is certainly a better alternative than alcohol or drugs.

Swami Mukundananda says, "Stress develops when we are attached to a particular outcome and are worried that things may not turn out as we desire." He says the remedy is simple enough: "Give up attachment to the outcome." How do we give up attachment to an outcome? Dr. Anna Kress, in her article, "3 Steps to Releasing Your Attachment to an Outcome," STR8 offers these suggestions:

> **Have compassion for the part of you that is attached to an outcome.**
> **Keep all options on the table**, even options that may not seem available.
> **Ask for more.** For example, if you are seeking a new job, imagine that you will have two or more good offers to choose from.

When learning a new skill, focusing intensely and being present to the activity at hand is excellent for reducing stress. When I started running and cycling, one of the first benefits I realized was stress reduction. Cycling in a group going 20 miles per hour and being only a few inches away from the other cyclists, or hiking at high altitudes through a boulder field, requires focus and presence. In those moments, I do not have the capacity to worry about work or sick parents or anything else; thus, my stress is reduced.

Interestingly, an activity can either be stressful or not, depending on how we look at it. I can take a stress reliever and turn it into a stressor. I like to get to the gym several days a week, which helps me manage my stress. However, sometimes just the challenge of getting to the gym is a stressor itself. At times, I remind myself that missing a workout is not the end of the world and may actually be good for me.

Choose the right amount of stress for your life. Too little or too much stress can shorten your life.

Sleep Seven Hours Per Night

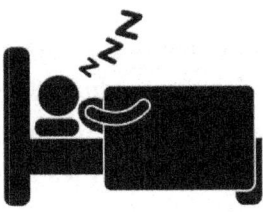

Sleep is essential for both brain health and physical health. Sleep is important in forming memories, learning, attention, being creative, and promoting fat loss.[SL1, SL2] Additionally, sleeping is thought to have a restorative function by facilitating the clearance of toxins that accumulate in the brain and nervous system. One such toxin is the protein, beta-amyloid, which is associated with Alzheimer's disease.[SL3]

Several studies have indicated a link between sleep deprivation and cardiovascular disease, type 2 diabetes, stroke, calcification of arteries, and chronic inflammation.[SL4, SL5] When sleep-deprived, the body produces fewer antibodies, which are needed to fight infection.[SL6]

A study of 1.1 million men and women from 30 to 102 years of age found that those with self-reported 6.5 to 7.4 hours of sleep had lower mortality rates than those with shorter or longer sleep durations. Seven hours of sleep per night was found to have the best survival rate, while those participants sleeping eight or more hours and those sleeping six or less hours were at increased risk of mortality.[SL7]

A study of 444 women agreed with the finding that shorter or longer sleep times lead to earlier mortality.[SL8] "Those with short or long sleep represented 42.4% of the sample and had two to four times greater mortality, corrected for multiple risk factors, compared to those with optimal sleep duration."

Sleep involves five phases, starting from light sleep and gradually moving to deep sleep and then on to rapid eye movement (REM) sleep. This cycle can repeat itself several times throughout the night. The duration for each phase is variable and changes throughout the course of the night, with more REM sleep happening later in the sleep cycle.[SL9] REM sleep gives rise to dreams, but excessive REM sleep has been associated with depression and feeling tired the following day.[SL10,] [SL11] Stress can extend REM sleep time. Consuming alcohol too close to bedtime lowers REM sleep time.

Melatonin is a hormone secreted by the pineal gland that has a sleep-promoting effect and a role in synchronizing the sleep-wake cycle.[SL12] Melatonin levels generally rise starting about two hours prior to a person's usual sleep time. Levels peak around 3 AM to 4 AM.[SL13] Melatonin also has a role in regulating body temperature and is an antioxidant found in high concentration in the mitochondria.[SL14] Melatonin production decreases as we age and melatonin supplementation can assist with sleeping.[SL15]

Sleep trackers are available for monitoring the duration and amount of time spent in each sleep phase. It is quite common and normal to wake up several times per night. On October 23 and October 24, 2019, I measured my sleep. Here is my data for the two nights:

Sleep Data for October 23 and 24, 2019

	October 23, 2019	October 24, 2019	Average
Total	7 Hr 53 Min	7 Hr 4 Min	7 Hr 28 Min
Actual	7 Hr 29 Min	6 Hr 38 Min	7 Hr 3 Min
Awake	22 Min	22 Min	22 Min
Light	4 Hr 33 Min	3 Hr 19 Min	3 Hr 56 Min
REM	2 Hr 44 Min	2 Hr 42 Min	2 Hr 43 Min
Deep	14 Min	41 Min	27 Min

If you want to improve your sleep, the National Sleep Foundation provides the following ideas:[SL16]

Avoid alcohol, cigarettes, and caffeine, including energy drinks.
Avoid large or spicy meals two hours before bedtime.
Avoid naps in the afternoon.
Exercise regularly, at any time of day.
Make your bedroom cool, quiet, and dark. Your bedroom should be between 60 and 67 degrees Fahrenheit. It should be free from noise,

including a partner's snoring. Earplugs, whitenoise machines, humidifiers, or fans may reduce disturbing noise. Blackout curtains or eye shades may help reduce light. **Sleep on a comfortable mattress and pillows. Use your bed mainly for sleep** to strengthen the association between bed and sleep. **Stick to a sleep schedule,** even on the weekends. **Wind down and practice a relaxing bedtime ritual an hour before bedtime. Maintain your circadian rhythms** by avoiding bright light in the evening and exposing yourself to sunlight in the morning. **Maintain a sleep diary** to expose sleep patterns or issues you may have. **Speak with your doctor or a sleep professional,** if needed.

Have you been burning the candle at both ends? Do you feel rested when you get up? Are there any steps you could take to improve your sleep? If so...

Take action to sleep seven hours every night.

Conclusion of the Longevity Best Practices

1 + 1 = 5

By combining two longevity pathways in roundworms, scientists were able to extend their lifespan by five times. This result surprised the researchers because the effects were highly synergistic. "The effect isn't one plus one equals two, it's one plus one equals five," said lead researcher, Jarod Rollins. The synergistic interaction may help explain why scientists have been unable to identify a single gene or approach responsible for living to an extraordinary old age.[CLB1] The roundworm research strongly suggests combinations of therapies are the most effective anti-aging protocols.

Implement as many of the longevity best practices as you can. Know your actions are synergistic and know your faith and beliefs are powerful and can overcome any obstacle.

Part III. Advanced Anti-Aging Techniques

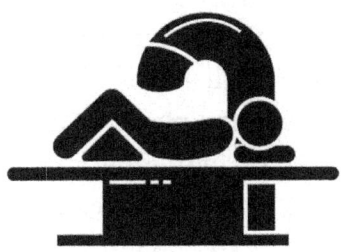

The best practices provide a solid foundation for longevity. They are available to us now and are readily accessible. Beyond these practices, there is reason to believe that advanced medical and anti-aging techniques will become available and will reduce or eliminate aging, rejuvenate damaged tissues and organs, and be personalized in ways that are inconceivable today.

Personalized Care

"Twenty-first-century medicine is becoming progressively proactive and has been described as predictive, personalized, preventive, and participatory medicine." [PC1]

According to the *Personalized Medicine Coalition*, "Personalized medicine is an evolving field in which physicians use diagnostic tests to determine which medical treatments will work best for each patient. By combining the data from those tests with an individual's medical history and circumstances, healthcare providers can develop targeted treatment and prevention plans."[PC2]

An article published by the American Academy of Anti-Aging Medicine suggests that, in the not too distant future, a one-size-fits-all approach to nutrition may be replaced with a nutrition plan that is customized for each person, based on individual characteristics, such as obvious ones like gender and age, as well as emerging understandings of DNA and our microbiome (gut bacteria).[PC3] The hope is that this personalized approach to nutrition could facilitate overall health, as well as help with prevention and management of diseases.

DNA testing has been around for a few years, with firms such as 23andMe offering ancestry and trait reports. Several years ago, I had my DNA analyzed for sports performance by *fitnessgenes.com*. The test involved taking a swab of cells from the inside of my cheek. They provided a report on about 50 of my sports and metabolism genes. The information was consistent with what I knew to be true. The report told me that my muscles are an even mix of fast and slow-twitch muscles, and I had genes that provided enhanced endurance. From these DNA results, the company offered customized meal and workout plans to optimize my athletic performance.

Platelet Rich Plasma (PRP) and Stem Cells

PRP injections are prepared by processing an extraction of a patient's blood to isolate and concentrate platelets.

Platelets, also called thrombocytes, are cells that form blood clots and perform other growth or healing functions. The provider injects a concentration of platelets into or near injured tissue (usually tendons, joints, or ligaments) to accelerate the healing process.[PRP1] Some, but not all, research studies related to PRP have shown beneficial results.

There are several types of stem cells,[PRP2] including:

Non-embryonic (adult) stem cells are a partially differentiated stem cell that can further differentiate to maintain and repair the tissue in which they are found. For example, neural stem cells are different from skin stem cells.

Induced pluripotent stem cells are adult stem cells that scientists have learned how to reset to an undifferentiated embryonic state.

Cord blood stem cells come from the umbilical cord of a new-born child.

Embryonic stem cells are unspecialized stem cells that can differentiate themselves and become tissue-specific cells with special functions.[PRP3] They are usually harvested from human embryos which has raised ethical issues. With the development of induced pluripotent stem cells, there is no or minimal need for embryonic stem cells.

The potential scope of stem cell therapies is large. Research is proceeding on stem cell therapies targeting the nervous system, heart tissue, teeth, orthopedics, and many more areas.

For example, Hematopoietic Stem Cell Transplantation (HSCT) is an approved therapy designed to reboot the immune system, which is responsible for damaging the brain and spinal cord in people with multiple sclerosis (MS).[PRP4] In HSCT, prior to chemotherapy treatment, blood cell-producing stem cells are collected and stored. After the patient's immune system has been depleted from chemotherapy drugs, the stored stem cells are reintroduced to the body. These stem cells, over time, reconstitute the immune system and (hopefully) do not continue to attack the brain and spinal cord, providing MS patients with relief.

During my triathlon season in 2012, I started to experience soreness in my left hip after my runs. Initially, the pain was minor and I did not address the issue that year. In October of 2013, I raced in a half marathon and did not perform as well as I had in the past. The next day I was not able to finish my run and I had to walk home because of my hip. I went to an orthopedist and was diagnosed with a torn labrum. I was offered a surgical procedure that could repair the labrum and involved a six-month recovery process. The other orthopedic option was a hip replacement.

As an alternative to orthopedic surgery, I investigated adult stem cell treatment. I was told that the results could be from none to complete recovery. I selected a stem cell treatment and PRP. The stem cell procedure involved extracting bone marrow from my hip and processing the marrow to collect the stem cells. These stem cells were then injected into the area near my torn labrum. These procedures did not allow me to return to regular running. However, I am almost 100% pain-free and I can do everything else, including walking, hiking, cycling, using the elliptical machine, and rock climbing. I am happy with this outcome.

Drugs and Supplements

The 2018 article, "Anti-Aging Drugs – Prospect of Longer Life?," suggests that rapamycin, metformin, resveratrol, and NAD precursors, such as NMN, are the most promising anti-aging drugs.[DS1] Mikhail V. Blagosklonny, MD, PhD, of the Roswell Park Comprehensive Cancer Center, states, "The overwhelming evidence suggests that rapamycin is a universal anti-aging drug – that is, it extends lifespan in all tested models from yeast to mammals, suppresses cell senescence and delays the onset of age-related diseases, which are manifestations of aging." He suggests that we need a holistic approach that implements controlled and monitored dosage of rapamycin, along with "the entire anti-aging recipe, including a complementary low carbohydrate diet and lifestyle changes." [DS2] Rapamycin is FDA approved only for a rare lung disease and to assist with kidney transplants in children. Some people are taking it "off-label", given its promise as an anti-aging compound.

Another promising class of anti-aging drugs is called senolytic drugs.[DS3] Non-cancerous cells normally stop dividing after about 50 or 60 cell divisions. A cell that stops dividing is called a senescent cell. Normally, the immune system detects and removes senescent cells. However, some senescent cells escape destruction by the immune system and cause problems. The accumulation of these cells is considered one of the root causes of aging.

Senolytic drugs target senescent cells and induce apoptosis (death) to these cells.[DS4] Animal studies of senolytic drugs have been promising and, as a result, pre-clinical trials with humans are proceeding. In the study, "The Clinical Potential of Senolytic Drugs," the authors conclude, "If senolytics or other interventions that target fundamental aging processes prove to be effective and safe in clinical trials, they could transform geriatric medicine by enabling prevention or treatment of multiple diseases and functional deficits in parallel, instead of one at a time." Initial results from a small trial using two senolytic drugs, dasatinib and quercetin have shown promise.[DS5] Unity Biotechnology and Oisín Biotechnologies are two of several companies focused on developing senolytic drugs.[DS6]

Other Approaches

A 2019 study from Harvard Medical School found that brains with more of a protein named REST were associated with longevity.[OA1, OA2] REST is responsible for dampening neural activity and protecting the brain.

What excited the researchers the most was that REST is associated with insulin and insulin-like growth factor 1. These signals are also associated with calorie restriction, which possibly helps humans live longer. Research with worms demonstrated that increasing REST increased their lifespan. Researchers agree that this is a promising area of study.[OA3]

In a 2019 article published in the *MIT Technology Review*, researcher Izpisúa Belmonte said he "believes epigenetic reprogramming may prove to be an 'elixir of life' that will extend human lifespan significantly." [OA4] Epigenetics determines whether a gene is activated or not. Epigenetic reprogramming is a way to reset the body's epigenetic markers and chemical switches that determine which genes are activated. Belmonte goes on to say that epigenetic reprogramming itself will not extend life indefinitely, but it could extend life by another 30 to 50 years. "I think the kid that will be living to 130 is already with us. He has already been born. I'm convinced."

Another promising area of research is three-dimensional bioprinting of cells and tissues. In September 2019, Harvard's Wyss Institute for Biologically Inspired Engineering announced a new technique called SWIFT (sacrificial writing into functional tissue) that could help produce "viable, organ-specific tissues with high cell density and function." [OA5] A group of researchers at Rensselaer Polytechnic Institute and Yale have printed skin that is complete with blood vessels.[OA6] Ultimately, they hope to be able to print skin, based on a patient's own DNA.

Scientist are applying Artificial intelligence (AI) to improve the health of humans. AI can assist with personalized medicine, drug development, augmenting physicians, and, potentially, much more. For example, a collaboration with Moorfields Eye Hospital, one of the best eye hospitals in the world, produced an AI application that could diagnose eye disease by analyzing detailed scans of the eye. The AI application performs as well as established doctors and it could be used anywhere. In theory, there is no limit to the type of problem that could be addressed with artificial intelligence.[OA7]

In January 2020, Microsoft launched a five-year, $40M health research program to address some of the world's medical challenges, using AI. The initiative will provide grants, data science experts, and technology focusing on three core areas:

> Accelerate research to prevent, diagnose, and treat diseases;

> Improve understanding of mortality and longevity to prepare for the next global health crisis; and

> Improve equity in healthcare.

This initiative is part of Microsoft's AI for Good, a $165M initiative to address societal challenges using advanced technologies.[OA8]

Advocacy Groups

Aubrey de Grey, PhD, with his research assistant, Michael Rae, wrote the book, *Ending Aging, The Rejuvenation Breakthroughs That Could Reverse Human Aging in Our Lifetime.*[AG1] This book introduces the idea that aging is a disease that can be eliminated by strategies that reverse the effects of aging on the human body.

de Grey also co-founded the Methuselah Foundation with David Gobel.[AG2] Their mission is to make "90 the new 50 by 2030." The foundation was named after Methuselah, of the Hebrew Bible, whose lifespan was recorded as 969 years. The Methuselah Foundation identifies six pathways for life extension:

New Parts for People – Being able to create replacement parts for our bodies.
Get the Crud Out – Removing harmful substances from both the cells and the organs of the body.
Restore the Rivers – Improve circulation.
Debug the Code – Returning cell function to a youthful state.
Restock the Shelves – Restocking stem cells of the immune system, the hypothalamus, and bone marrow.

Lust for Life – Ability and desire to live because of increased health.The Methuselah Foundation website says, "We incubate and sponsor mission-relevant ventures, fund research, and support projects and prizes, to accelerate breakthroughs in longevity."

Exponential Medicine is bringing together clinicians, innovators, investors, and executives, to explore game-changing health and medical technologies.[AG3] Founded in 2011, Exponential Medicine is "focused on the implications of breakthrough developments such as 3D printing, personalized stem cell lines, point-of-care lab-on-a-chip diagnostics, robotics, augmented intelligence, machine learning, large-scale bioinformatics, synthetic biology, low-cost genomics, gene editing, blockchain, and more."

The mission of the *Regenerative Medicine Foundation* is "to accelerate regenerative medicine to improve health and deliver cures." [AG4] They sponsor events and recognize leaders in the field of regenerative medicine. They advocate for patients, promoting the delivery of new treatments and cures. The foundation also supports regulations for regenerative medicine.

The mission of the *American Academy of Anti-Aging Medicine* (A4M) is to advance tools, technology, and transformations in healthcare that can detect, treat, and prevent diseases associated with aging. A4M is also dedicated to educating healthcare professionals, practitioners, and scientists.[AG5] "We're not about growing old gracefully," said Dr. Ronald Klatz, of A4M. *Fight Aging!* encourages "the development of medical technologies, lifestyles, and other means that will help people live comfortably, healthily, and capable, for as long as they desire, well beyond the current limits of mortality." Their website is a great source of information related to aging science, research, therapies, and advocacy.[AG6]

Conclusion of Advanced Anti-Aging Techniques

Given the amount of research and development currently underway, I believe novel procedures that can slow down or reverse aging will emerge quickly. Of course, we do not need to know that any of these advanced treatments are being developed and will be available to us in the future, unless we think we do.

Having faith that advanced anti-aging treatments are coming may induce a powerful placebo effect that could be more valuable than the treatments themselves.

Part IV. Reasons for Hope and Optimism

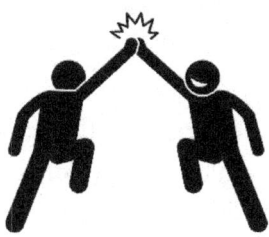

I believe there are many reasons for hope and optimistic. Even though not everyone on the planet is on board yet, there are forces at work that are driving us to a clean, sustainable economy that can be accessed and benefitted by everyone. There are plenty of problems and plenty of things that could go terribly wrong, including COVID-19, yet I believe that they will not hold us back for long. With our resourcefulness and technology, we will adapt quickly.

Large companies, such as Walmart and Ford, have been driving sustainability initiatives through their companies and supply chains. Initially, Walmart struggled with the definition of sustainability.[RHO1] This led Walmart and other companies to form the Sustainability Consortium in 2009 to "drive positive environmental and social change within the consumer goods industry." [RHO2] Their goal is "to create a planet where the resources we use to create the products we consume have a neutral effect on our world."

How many people can the earth support? Can it even sustainably support our current population? Many studies have considered this question. Not surprisingly, the study results vary considerably depending upon the assumptions and desired outcomes. Some studies indicate a carrying capacity of the planet of one billion people or less while other studies conclude that a capacity of 16 billion or more people is possible.[RHO3] Obviously, to double our current population would put significant pressure on the planet but, I believe, if we create a sustainable, sharing economy, it could be possible. Simply improving our collective health could save billions in healthcare costs. A study suggests that delaying death could have a net benefit to society of greater than $7 trillion.[RHO4] The results of this study suggest that these benefits would compound and "extend to future generations."

Jeremy Rifkin, the author of *The Zero Marginal Cost Society*, [RHO5] points to several aspects of our economy that are already free and others that are headed that way. Many information services have been free for some time. This includes email, data storage, and office applications. Increasingly, access to information is becoming free. As an extension of information, online education is headed in the same direction. The future of education does not look like large campuses housing students in remote areas. The future of education looks to be online, virtual, and local. A study of history using virtual reality would bring alive the past. Imagine being able to experience ancient Rome or Egypt using virtual reality.

Energy provided by the wind and sun is driving the marginal cost of energy to zero. The race is on to harvest the cleanest, most abundant energy with the minimum upfront investment and ongoing costs. Different approaches include nuclear fusion, advanced nuclear fission techniques such as liquid fluoride thorium reactors, tidal, and advanced solar technology, including space-based solar energy. Thorium-based nuclear reactors would be much safer and cleaner than conventional uranium, light water reactors. Fusion and fission reactions require fuel and would not be zero marginal cost, but any one of these advances could be game-changing for the planet and accelerate the pace of electrification and development for everyone.

Our current methods of mass production of food are both inefficient and wasteful. Peter Diamandis, founder of the X-Prize and Singularity University, points to vertical farms as one of the potential solutions that can lower food transportation costs and water demands.[RHO6] Vertical farming is where food is grown in "vertical stacks, in skyscrapers and buildings, rather than outside in fields." The precise amount of water, light, and nutrients can be delivered to maximize the plants' growing needs and lower the overall cost and environmental impact.

Another potentially impactful food innovation is cultured meat. Cultured meat is meat that is grown from "a few cells into a full-blown meal." [RHO7] Meat production is disastrous to the health of the planet. Just considering water, meat production consumes 70% of global water resources. It is estimated that cultured meat could use "99% less land, 82% to 96% less water, and produce 78% to 96% less greenhouse gases." Even a small shift of meat production to cultured meat would provide considerable relief to the planet. Would you want to eat cultured meat? It might be a healthier solution. Perhaps, in the not too distant future, hamburgers will actually be good for us, provided the product contains essential vitamins and high-quality protein with reduced saturated fats.

Automated, self-driving vehicles will reduce traffic congestion and transportation-related deaths. The Association for Safe International Road Travel reports that over one million people die in road crashes each year.[RHO8] Electrification and automation of transportation will have many other benefits, including improved productivity and less need for vehicle parking in confined cities.[RHO9] Futurist Thomas Fry believes that any fears related to self-driving vehicles will be short-lived.

Governments are also getting on board with the changes brought about by longer lifespans as they are starting to revise and adapt their policies and programs. In Singapore, the government is investing $3 billion, "to support lifelong learning and employability, health and wellness, financial literacy, and multi-generational housing among other initiatives." [RHO10]

Part V. Afterword

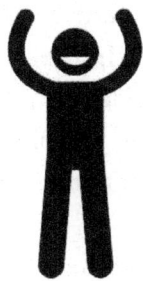

In this book, I discuss 17 best practices to live a long, happy, and meaningful life. The practices are common sense, but they are unique compared to other longevity books because I have included concepts of belief and spirituality and have organized the practices into categories of spirit, body, and mind. I have also included my experiences and stories. I hope my stories have been helpful and, perhaps, inspired you.

I believe that there is synergy in performing several of the best practices simultaneously. I am sure you noticed that diet and exercise are a component in almost all of the body and mind best practices. To provide a simplistic example, eating a healthy diet can lead to weight loss and then to better self-esteem, which can lead to better sleep, which can lead to helping others.

For most people, decisions related to implementing the best practices are a matter of choice, and choices are driven by beliefs. Have any of your beliefs been challenged by this book?

I strongly believe what we do for other people is just as important as what we do for ourselves, and the best way for us to get what we want is to help others get what they want. Those we help may support us, and we establish a virtuous cycle of care and support. Do you agree that helping other people is the best way to achieve what you want to achieve?

My intention is to make the information and techniques accessible and available to anyone who is interested. Most of these techniques are not expensive. With the exception of aesthetics, the spirit-based best practices have minimal cost. I choose to spend about $2,000 per year on cosmetic treatments. I spend about $2,000 per year on supplements and another $500 per year on hormone treatments and testing. I also purchase a $250 blood panel every year. I purchase healthy food and I have a gym membership. I believe that healthy eating is not more expensive than eating junk food, and a gym membership is not required for moving your body.

By contrast, I was invited to a group focusing on advanced anti-aging strategies that required a $50,000 admission fee. The fee was for access to information and people, not for a single product or service. I can only imagine how much the services they are offering cost.

If we believe and help each other we can all live well beyond 120 years, be happy and have meaningful lives. I am suggesting that we can have it all. We are all one. There is enough for everyone. I choose to help as many people as I can because I know that helping others will also help me.

Afterword

The way I look at this, we are in a no-lose situation. My life is not going to be worse off for helping other people live longer, better lives even if I receive nothing in return. While there is not much to lose, there is, potentially, a lot to be gained. I can see myself helping many people living better lives, including helping some people in poverty improve their standard of living.

What are you going to do as a result of reading this book? If you are not sure, the chapter, "Apply the Best Practices to Your Life," provides you a tool to inventory your current situation and to think of ways of improving your life.

What do you have to lose?

What I would like is to hear from you. Please join me in the conversation at *www.livewellbeyond120.com*.

Part VI. Afterword, COVID-19

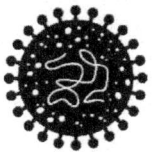

This book was in the process of final edits in March 2020 when the COVID-19 pandemic swept across the planet. Initially, I was not sure if my book would be relevant during and after the pandemic subsides. After re-reading my text, I decided to move forward with the book. I added a few comments within the text and this additional chapter.

There are still many reasons for hope and optimism, perhaps even more so in the wake of the pandemic. The pandemic is not species-ending. Most people are going to survive this event. I am not attempting to minimize the loss of life. The potential impacts brought by the disease and how we responded to it are a disturbing thought. In particular, it is frightening to think of how the poor and underdeveloped countries, especially those with large centralized populations like Kenya, will be impacted.

For the first time in human history, we have an event that affects everyone. COVID-19 does not respect national borders and no place on the planet is safe from COVID-19. I believe it is inevitable that the world's political community will come together in some form. The solution to COVID-19 must be global before we can return to a new normal. The U.S. cannot be healthy if Mexico or India or even Thailand is not. The head of the United Nations World Health Organization is asking for this to begin through the G20, the world's 20 richest nations.[AC1]

I believe that once we do come together and solve the COVID-19 crisis, there will be a larger conversation around how to deal with problems of poverty, sustainability, and lack of governmental transparency. The solutions will be good for everyone. The irony is that communities will need to become more self-sufficient and global at the same time.

In addition, I hope the religious leaders of the world will unite as well. I would not be surprised to see Pope Francis reach out to the Dali Lama and other religious leaders for joint prayer and meditation services. This process could have an important healing function.

Either political or spiritual unification, even briefly, could rankle those who resist change, but change will come because what we were doing before was not working well enough for enough people.

Many people will live long, happy, and meaningful lives during and after COVID-19. Until the new normal emerges, there will be challenges and difficult times. However, CWG suggests that we see the perfection of everything. We are fortunate that we have unique opportunities to express who we really are. We live in interesting times for sure.

Part VII. Apply the Best Practices to Your Life

It's your turn now. I encourage you to take a few moments to consider each of the longevity best practices.

Start with your current age and assessments of your biological age and life expectancy.

Your current age	
Your RealAge® as determined by *sharecare.com*	
Additional years you can expect to live from the Social Security Life Expectancy Calculator	
Life expectancy from the BLUE ZONES® True Vitality Test	
Were you surprised by the results of the calculators? How?	

Complete your current status and rank yourself, with 1 being the worst rating possible and 10 being the best that you think is possible by anyone.

Spirit-Based Longevity Best Practices	Questions to Consider Asking Yourself	Self-Rating (1 to 10)	Current Status
Have Positive Beliefs of Longevity	How long are you going to live? Why are you going to live to the age you identified? What are your beliefs about life? (Is life good?) How do you feel about the future? Are you optimistic? (Consider performing a belief inventory.)		
Have a Faith or Spiritual Practice	Do you have a regular spiritual practice? What is it? Are you comfortable with your practice? Are you open to the ideas of others?		

Pray or Meditate	Do you pray or meditate? What form of prayer or meditation do you use? How long do you pray or meditate? How often do you pray or meditate? How do you feel after you pray or meditate?		
Have Healthy Relation-ships	Do you love yourself? What are your best intimate, family, friend, co-worker relationships? What are your weakest relationships? Why?		
Be Purposeful and Service-Oriented	What is your purpose? Are you of service to others in your work, in your community?		
Be Present and Happy	How often are you happy or sad? When are you happy? How often are you present? (list those times)		

Use Aesthetics to Feel Better and Live Longer	How do you feel about how you look? Do you utilize aesthetics or cosmetics to improve the way you look? If not, why not? Have you thought about a cosmetic procedure and did not do it?		

Body-Based Longevity Best Practices

Have a Health Plan	Do you believe your health is your responsibility and are you being proactive about it? Do you have a team of healthcare professionals who you work with and trust? (Doctors, dentists, physical therapists, personal trainers, health coaches) When is the last time you saw them? Do they know your goals? Do you have a plan? Do you have access to the healthcare system?		

Eat a Natural Diet	What is strong is your diet? How many calories do you take in? What is your percentage of protein, carbohydrates, and fat? (Many people overestimate the quality of their diet. Consider recording a food diary for three days.)		
Consider Taking Basic Supple-ments	What supplements are you currently taking? What doses? (List out) Why are you taking them?		
Move Your Body	Do you feel fit? How often and how do you move your body? (How many steps per day do you take?) What do you like to do? Does your current physical condition limit your activities?		

Maintain Healthy Body Compo- sition	Determine your body mass index by using an online BMI calculator. What range is your BMI? Obtain a measurement of your body fat percentage. What range is your body fat?		
Optimize Your Hormones	Do you know your hormone levels (do not expect insurance to pay for this)? Have you discussed your hormones levels with your doctor?		
Avoid Toxic Substances	Have you been or are you exposed to toxic substances (at work, at home)? Which ones and how much is your exposure?		

Mind-Based Longevity Best Practices

Protect Your Brain	What do you do to nurture your brain?		

Choose the Right Amount of Stress	How much stress do you have in your life, in your job, in your relationships, in your health? Are you bored? Are you overwhelmed? How well do you manage your stress?		
Sleep Seven Hours Per Night	How much sleep do you get? Is it restful? Does your partner keep you awake?		

Now, based on your current status, list your ideas for improvement for each of the best practices. Where you ranked yourself low, why was that? What can you do to improve those practices?

Spirit-Based Longevity Best Practices	Questions to Consider Asking Yourself	Improvement Ideas

Have Positive Beliefs of Longevity	What are your core beliefs? (Did you perform a belief inventory?) Do your beliefs limit you? How could you improve your beliefs? Take one or more of the Implicit Association Tests to learn about your biases.	
Have a Faith or Spiritual Practice	Does your practice reflect your truths and beliefs? (Often people adopt the belief systems of others without giving it much thought.) Are you open to the idea of a spiritual practice if you do not have one? What else could you do to improve your faith or spiritual practice?	

Pray or Meditate	Are you praying or meditating frequently or long enough? Do you feel that your prayer or meditation is effective? Are you open to different modes of prayer or meditation? Is there a prayer or meditation group that you could join?	
Have Healthy Relation-ships	Is your relationship to yourself healthy? How can you have more healthy relationships? What can you do to improve your existing relationships? Would having a pet improve your well-being?	

Be Purposeful and Service-Oriented	Are you comfortable with your purpose? If not, do you have a plan to find your purpose? Is your service satisfying to you? What calling or mission is important to you? What service could you do to improve the life of someone else?	
Be Present and Happy	Regarding the things that make you happy, describe why they make you happy? What could you do more of to be happier? When you are present in the moment of your experience what captures your interest?	
Use Aesthetics to Feel Better and Live Longer	What cosmetics or aesthetics are you going to consider (none is ok if you know why)?	

Body-Based Longevity Best Practices

Have a Health Plan	Do you have an idea of how to create a health plan if you need one? Do you need to change doctors?	
Eat a Natural Diet	Did you keep a food diary? Do you know what needs to improve? Are you motivated to improve your diet? (If not, why not)? Do you need help creating a proper diet for yourself?	
Consider Taking Basic Supple-ments	Do you need assistance with determining what supplements and doses would be right for you?	

Move Your Body	Do you know what you need to do to improve your physical health? (Identify those changes) Are you motivated to make changes? Would assistance, coaching, or accountability help you?	
Maintain Healthy Body Composition	If your BMI is not in the healthy range, do you acknowledge you need to make changes? Do you know how to make changes to improve your body composition?	
Optimize Your Hormones	If you do not know your hormone levels, get them measured through a diagnostic. If your hormones are not in normal ranges, what, in conjunction with your doctor, are you doing about it?	
Avoid Toxic Substances	What can you do to eliminate or reduce your exposure to toxic substances?	

Mind-Based Longevity Best Practices

Protect Your Brain	What steps can you take to help prevent brain diseases such as Alzheimer's? What else can you do to stimulate your brain?	
Choose the Right Amount of Stress	What steps can you take to manage your stress better (move closer to work, change jobs, etc.)? If you are bored, what can you do to stimulate yourself?	
Sleep Seven Hours Per Night	What steps can you take to improve your sleep? Can you keep better hours? Can you improve your bedding or your bedroom? Would earplugs or an eye mask help? Would controlling your partner's snoring help you?	

To provide an example, here is what my table looks like:

Spirit-Based Longevity Best Practices	Current Status	Self-Rating (1 to 10)	Improvement Ideas
Have Positive Beliefs of Longevity	I am living well beyond 120. My cells age only every other day.	8	Continue to develop additional positive beliefs about life and longevity.
Have a Faith or Spiritual Practice	Regularly attending church.	7	Learn about other faiths and adopt what feels right to me.
Pray or Meditate	I see the value of daily meditation and am a regular practitioner.	8	Learn about additional styles of meditation and look for other group meditation opportunities.
Have Healthy Relation-ships	I have a few high-quality relationships, personally and with friends and family.	6	Continue to focus on high-quality relationships and see the goodness in all people.

Be Purposeful and Service-Oriented	My mission is to help as many people as I can to live long, happy, and meaningful lives.	7	Look for ways to have a large impact on hunger and poverty.
Be Present and Happy	I have made many changes to be more present in my day-to-day life. My gratitude helps me be happy.	7	Continue to find and be present to the beauty of everything around me.
Use Aesthetics to Feel Better and Live Longer	Minimal with BOTOX® and some hair color.	7	Stay open to different opportunities with good cost-benefit and risk-reward ratios.

Body-Based Longevity Best Practices

Have a Health Plan	I meet with my primary doctor annually. I meet with other specialists as needed.	7	Share my goals with all my healthcare providers. Change doctors as needed.
Eat a Natural Diet	My diet is solidly healthy, but I do eat some protein bars and corn chips.	8	Rely more on plant-based, natural foods.

Consider Taking Basic Supplements	I consume a wide variety of supplements. See corresponding chapter in this book for specifics.	8	Continue to research efficacy and cost-effectiveness of supplements.
Move Your Body	I exercise six days per week, alternating three days of weights and three days of cardio.	8	Set some great goals for when I turn 60. Use a coach more often. Get more massages.
Maintain Healthy Body Composition	My BMI is 23.4, which is in the healthy range.	9	Continue to monitor.
Optimize Your Hormones	I am currently taking testosterone and anastrozole (minimizes the conversion of testosterone to estrogen).	8	Continue to monitor.
Avoid Toxic Substances	I am conscious of avoiding toxic substances. I am unfortunately exposed to plastics in particular.	9	Reduce exposure to plastics, especially from cooking food in a microwave oven.

Mind-Based Longevity Best Practices

Protect Your Brain	I have learned to play guitar recently. I am taking fish oil and acetyl-l-carnitine.	8	Engage in more nature experiences.
Choose the Right Amount of Stress	I have generally avoided excessive stress.	8	Look for additional ways to measure and reduce stress.
Sleep Seven Hours Per Night	I usually get 6.5 to 7.5 hours of sleep per night.	8	Monitor and look for ways to improve sleep quality.

Part VIII. References

Your Cells Are Listening

YCL1 Carroll, Lee. "End of Disease Inheritance." *Kryon,* 2019, audio.kryon.com/en/Disease inheritance-Kauai-6.mp3. Accessed 2 February 2020.

YCL2 Carroll, Lee. "Invisible Things Part 3." *Kryon, 2019,* audio.kryon.com/en/Invisible Things P3.mp3. Accessed 2 February 2020.

YCL3 Walsch, Neale Donald. *Conversations with God, Book 4: Awaken the Species.* Rainbow Ridge Books. 2017.

How Long We Live

HLL1 Arias, Elizabeth and Xu, Jiaquan. "United States Life Tables, 2017." *CDC National Vital Statistics Report,* vol. 68, no. 7, June 24, 2019. www.cdc.gov/nchs/data/nvsr/nvsr68/nvsr68_07-508.pdf. Accessed 2 February 2020.

HLL2 "Life Expectancy for Countries." *Info Please,* 11 January 2020, www.infoplease.com/world/health-and-social-statistics/life-expectancy-countries-0. Accessed 2 February 2020.

HLL3 Valdez, Carlos. "123-year-old Bolivian man is oldest living person ever documented." *NBC News,* 16 August 2013, www.nbcnews.com/news/world/123-year-old-bolivian-man-oldest-living-person-ever-documented-flna6C10934840. Accessed 2 February 2020.

HLL4 Young, Robert and Adams, John M. "Validated Deceased Supercentenarians." *Gerontology Research*

Group, 1 February 2020, supercentenarian-research-foundation.org/TableE.aspx. Accessed 2 February 2020.

HLL5 Purdom, Georgia and Menton, David. "Did People Like Adam and Noah Really Live Over 900 Years of Age?" *Answers In Genesis*, 27 May 2010, answersingenesis.org/bible-timeline/genealogy/did-adam-and-noah-really-live-over-900-years. Accessed 2 February 2020.

HLL6 Walsch, Neale Donald. *The Complete Conversations with God: An Uncommon Dialogue*. Penguin Publishing Group. Kindle Edition.

HLL7 Gertrude Cecelia Schnelker Weber was born 28 November 1912 and died 15 January 2013.

HLL8 "Retirement & Survivors Benefits: Life Expectancy Calculator." *Social Security Administration*, www.ssa.gov/OACT/population/longevity.html. Accessed 2 February 2020.

HLL9 "The True Vitality Test™." *BLUE ZONES®*, apps.bluezones.com/en/vitality. Accessed 2 February 2020.

Our Beliefs About Health and Longevity

BAL1 "The power of the placebo effect." *Harvard Medical School, Harvard Health Publishing*, 9 August 2019, www.health.harvard.edu/mental-health/the-power-of-the-placebo-effect. Accessed 2 February 2020.

BAL2 Gholipour, Bahar. "Placebo Effect May Account for Half of Drug's Efficacy." *Live Science*, 8 January 2014, www.livescience.com/42430-placebo-effect-half-of-drug-efficacy.html. Accessed 2 February 2020.

BAL3 Brynie, Faith. "The Placebo Effect: How It Works." *Psychology Today*, 10 January 2020, www.psychologytoday.com/us/blog/brain-sense/201201/the-placebo-effect-how-it-works. Accessed 2 February 2020.

BAL4 Emanuel, Ezekiel J. "Why I Hope to Die at 75." *The Atlantic*, October 2014, www.theatlantic.com/magazine/archive/2014/10/why-i-hope-to-die-at-75/379329. Accessed 2 February 2020.

BAL5 Olesen, Jacob. "Fear of Getting Old Phobia – Gerascophobia." *FEAROF.NET*, www.fearof.net/fear-of-getting-old-phobia-gerascophobia. Accessed 2 February 2020.

BAL6 "Living to 120 and Beyond: Americans' Views on Aging, Medical Advances and Radical Life Extension." *Pew Research Center, Religion and Public Life*, 6 August 2013, www.pewforum.org/2013/08/06/living-to-120-and-beyond-americans-views-on-aging-medical-advances-and-radical-life-extension. Accessed 2 February 2020.

BAL7 Palmer, Brian. "I Wish I Was a Little Bit Shorter. The research is clear: Being tall is hazardous to your health." *Slate*, 30 July 2013, slate.com/technology/2013/07/height-and-longevity-the-research-is-clear-being-tall-is-hazardous-to-your-health.html. Accessed 2 February 2020.

BAL8 Herskind, A. M., et al. "The heritability of human longevity: a population-based study of 2872 Danish twin pairs born 1870-1900." *Human Genetics*, vol. 97,3 (1996): 319-23. doi:10.1007/bf02185763.

Living 120 Years Is Like Running a Four-Minute Mile

FMM1 "No detectable limit to how long people can live." *McGill,* 28 June 2017, www.mcgill.ca/newsroom/channels/news/no-detectable-limit-how-long-people-can-live-268769. Accessed 2 February 2020.

FMM2 Marck Adrien, Antero Juliana, Berthelot Geoffroy, Saulière Guillaume, Jancovici Jean-Marc, Masson-Delmotte Valérie, Boeuf Gilles, Spedding Michael, Le Bourg Éric and Toussaint Jean-François. "Are We Reaching the Limits of Homo Sapiens?" *Frontiers in Physiology,* vol. 8. www.frontiersin.org/article/10.3389/fphys.2017.00812. doi:10.3389/fphys.2017.00812. 2017.

Research That Influenced My Knowledge and Beliefs About Longevity

RBL1 Walford, Roy L. *The 120-Year Diet: How to Double Your Vital Years.* Simon & Schuster (0p) ISBN 978-0-671-46677-0.

RBL2 "Biosphere II Project." *Encyclopedia.com,* 3 February 2020, www.encyclopedia.com/science-and-technology/biology-and-genetics/environmental-studies/biosphere-ii-project. Accessed 2 February 2020.

RBL3 Dhahbi, Joseph M., Kim, Hyon-Jeen, Mote, Patricia L., Beaver, Robert J., Spindler, Stephen R. "Temporal linkage between the phenotypic and genomic responses to caloric restriction." *Proceedings of the National Academy of Sciences,* Apr 2004, 101 (15) 5524-5529. doi:

10.1073/pnas.0305300101.
www.pnas.org/content/101/15/5524

RBL4 "Caloric restriction mimetic." *Wikipedia.*
en.wikipedia.org/wiki/Caloric_restriction_mimetic.
Accessed 2 February 2020.

RBL5 "7 Health Benefits of Resveratrol Supplements."
Healthline.
www.healthline.com/nutrition/resveratrol#section7.
Accessed 2 February 2020.

RBL6 Das, Abhirup, et al. "Impairment of an Endothelial
NAD+-H2S Signaling Network Is a Reversible Cause of
Vascular Aging." *Cell*, vol. 173, ISSUE 1, P74-89.E20,
MARCH 22, 2018/doi: 10.1016/j.cell.2018.02.008.
https://www.cell.com/cell/fulltext/S0092-
8674(18)30152-1

RBL7 Yaku, Keisuke, et al. "NAD Metabolism in Cancer
Therapeutics." *Frontiers in Oncology*, vol. 8 622, 12
December 2018. doi:10.3389/fonc.2018.00622.
https://www.frontiersin.org/articles/10.3389/fonc.2018
.00622/full.

RBL8 Ehninger D, Neff F, and Xie K. "Longevity,
aging and rapamycin." *Cell Mol Life Sci.* 2014;71:4325–
46. doi: 10.1007/s00018-014-1677-1.

RBL9 Somers, Suzanne. *Bombshell: Explosive Medical
Secrets That Will Redefine Aging.* Harmony. 2012.

RBL10 "Suzanne Somers's Quest to Educate the World
About How to Delay Aging." *Life Extension Foundation,*
June 2012,
www.lifeextension.com/magazine/2012/6/suzanne-

somers-quest-to-educate-world-about-how-to-delay-aging. Accessed 2 February 2020.

RBL11 Buettner, Dan. *The Blue Zones: 9 Lessons for Living Longer From the People Who've Lived the Longest.* 2nd ed. Washington, D.C.: National Geographic, 2012.

RBL12 Cao Z, Wang R, Cheng Y, Yang H, Li S, Sun L, Xu W, Wang Y. "Adherence to a healthy lifestyle counteracts the negative effects of risk factors on all-cause mortality in the oldest-old." *Aging* (Albany NY). 2019, 11:7605-7619. doi: 10.18632/aging.102274, www.aging-us.com/article/102274/text

My Spiritual Transformation

MST1 Walsch, Neale Donald. *The Complete Conversations with God: An Uncommon Dialogue.* Penguin Publishing Group. Kindle Edition.

MST2 "Luke 6:31." *Esv: Study Bible: English Standard Version.* Wheaton, Ill: Crossway Bibles, 2007.

MST3 Walsch, Neale Donald. *Conversations with God, Book 4: Awaken the Species.* Rainbow Ridge Books. Kindle Edition.

We Are All In This Together

ALL1 Lawrence, Andrew. "How Sterling K. Brown Plans to Live to 100." *Men's Health,* 15 October 2020, www.menshealth.com/entertainment/a29413239/sterling-k-brown-age-longevity-interview. Accessed 3 February 2020.

ALL2 Distel, Jan Rose. "'I'm going to live to be 110 years old!' Suzanne Somers, 67, talks life after breast cancer and reveals how she stays healthy in new Closer interview." *Boomer Chick*, 26 September 2014, www.boomerchickuniverse.com/im-going-to-live-to-be-110-years-old-suzanne-somers-67-talks-life-after-breast-cancer-and-reveals-how-she-stays-healthy-in-new-closer-interview. Accessed 3 February 2020.

ALL3 Taylor, Chris. "The End of Aging. Harvard's genetics genius says we can live past 120 with supplements and lifestyle tweaks. Prepare to meet your future descendants." *Mashable*, 2019, mashable.com/feature/aging. Accessed February 3, 2020.

ALL4 "Population ageing and development: Ten years after Madrid." *United Nations*, Department of Economic and Social Affairs, Population Division, Population Facts, No. 2012/4, December 2012, www.un.org/en/development/desa/population/public ations/pdf/popfacts/popfacts_2012-4.pdf. Accessed 3 February 2020.

ALL5 Kennedy, Pagan. "The Secret to a Longer Life? Don't Ask These Dead Longevity Researchers." *New York Times*, 9 March 2019, www.nytimes.com/2018/03/09/opinion/sunday/longe vity-pritikin-atkins.html. Accessed 3 February 2020.

Have Positive Beliefs of Longevity

PBL1 "Transforming the Workforce for Children Birth Through Age 8. A Unifying Foundation." *Institute of Medicine*; Board on Children, Youth, and Families, Allen, LaRue, and Kelly, Bridget B., Editors. National Academies Press. 23 July 2015.

PBL2 Brenner, Abigail. "The Belief Inventory. What do you believe?" *Psychology Today*, 13 December 2013, www.psychologytoday.com/us/blog/influx/201312/the-belief-inventory. Accessed 3 February 2020.

PBL3 "Project Implicit." implicit.harvard.edu/implicit/takeatest.html. Accessed 3 February 2020.

PBL4 Vedantam, Shankar. "See No Bias. Many Americans believe they are not prejudiced. Now a new test provides powerful evidence that a majority of us really are." *Washington Post*, p. W12, 23 January 2005, www.washingtonpost.com/wp-dyn/articles/A27067-2005Jan21.html. Accessed 3 February 2020.

Have a Faith or Spiritual Practice

FSP1 Wallace, L. E., Anthony, R., End, C. M., & Way, B. M. (2019). "Does Religion Stave Off the Grave? Religious Affiliation in One's Obituary and Longevity." *Social Psychological and Personality Science*, 10(5), 662–670. doi:10.1177/1948550618779820

FSP2 Pullella, Philip and Eljechtimi, Ahmed. "Conversion is not your mission, pope tells Catholics in Morocco." *Reuters*, 31 March 2019, www.reuters.com/article/us-pope-morocco/conversion-is-not-your-mission-pope-tells-catholics-in-morocco-idUSKCN1RC0EI. Accessed 3 February 2020.

FSP3 Beseme, Sarah, et al. "Transcriptional Changes in Cancer Cells Induced by Exposure to a Healing Method." *Dose-Response*, July 2018. doi:10.1177/1559325818782843.

Pray or Meditate

POM1 Mead, Elaine. "The History and Origin of Meditation." *Positive Psychology*, 17 January 2020, positivepsychology.com/history-of-meditation. Accessed 3 February 2020.

POM2 "What is Prayer?" *Billy Graham Evangelical Association*, 1 June 2004, billygraham.org/answer/what-is-prayer. Accessed 3 February 2020.

POM3 Thorpe, Matthew, "12 Science-Based Benefits of Meditation." *Healthline*, 5 July 2017, www.healthline.com/nutrition/12-benefits-of-meditation. Accessed 3 February 2020.

POM4 Thorpe, Matthew, "Promotes Emotional Health." *Healthline*, 5 July 2017, www.healthline.com/nutrition/12-benefits-of-meditation#section3. Accessed 3 February 2020.

POM5 Dienstmann, Giovanni. "76 Benefits of Meditation and Mindfulness (Scientific Research)." *Live & Dare*, 2015, liveanddare.com/benefits-of-meditation. Accessed 3 February 2020.

POM6 Juergens, Jeffrey. "The Purpose of the 12 Steps." *Addiction Center*, 5 December 2019, www.addictioncenter.com/treatment/12-step-programs. Accessed 3 February 2020.

POM7 Admin. "Alcoholics Anonymous Step 11: Commit to a Spiritual Practice." *Recovery.Org, American Addiction Centers*, 7 December 2018, www.recovery.org/alcoholics-anonymous/step-11. Accessed 3 February 2020.

POM8 "Meditation, Stress, and Your Health." *WebMD*, Ratini, Melinda Reviewer, 18 June 2018, www.webmd.com/balance/guide/meditation-natural-remedy-for-insomnia#2. Accessed 3 February 2020.

POM9 Rhodes, Tricia McCary. "Types of Prayer." *Prayer Online*, www.prayeronline.org.au/types-of-prayer. Accessed 3 February 2020.

POM10 "Types of meditation." *Headspace*, www.headspace.com/meditation/techniques. Accessed 3 February 2020.

POM11 "The technique for inner peace and wellness." *Transcendental Meditation®*, TM.org. Accessed 3 February 2020.

POM12 "What is Qigong?" *Qigong Institute*, qigonginstitute.org. Accessed 3 February 2020.

POM13 Winter, Theo. "Evidence for Mindfulness: A Research Summary for the Corporate Sceptic." *Association for Talent Development*, 25 March 2016, www.td.org/insights/evidence-for-mindfulness-a-research-summary-for-the-corporate-sceptic. Accessed 3 February 2020.

POM14 Manciagli, Dana. "Benefits of Meditation in the Workplace." *Arizona State University, Thunderbird School of Global Management*, 29 November 2017, thunderbird.asu.edu/knowledge-network/benefits-meditation-workplace. Accessed 3 February 2020.

POM15 Grover Jr., MD, Fred. *Spiritual Genomics*. Spiritual Genomics Press. 2019.

POM16 Conklin, Quinn, et al. "Telomere lengthening after three weeks of an intensive insight meditation retreat." *Psychoneuroendocrinology*, 61, 26-7. doi:10.1016/j.psyneuen.2015.07.462.

POM17 "Researchers discover that the rate of telomere shortening predicts species lifespan." *The Spanish National Cancer Research Centre*, 8 July 2018, phys.org/news/2019-07-telomere-shortening-species-lifespan.html. Accessed 23 March 2020.

POM18 Lazar, Sara W., et al. "Meditation experience is associated with increased cortical thickness." *Neuroreport*, vol. 16,17 (2005): 1893-7. doi:10.1097/01.wnr.0000186598.66243.19

Have Healthy Relationships

HHR1 "Do Social Ties Affect Our Health? Exploring the Biology of Relationships." *National Institute of Health, News In Health*, February 2017, newsinhealth.nih.gov/2017/02/do-social-ties-affect-our-health. Accessed 3 February 2020.

HHR2 Roy, Sandip. "How To Love Yourself Without Guilt." Happiness India Project, happyproject.in/love-yourself. Accessed 3 February 2020.

HHR3 Davey-Smith, G., et al. "Sex and Death: Are They Related? Findings for the Caerphilly Cohort Study." *BMJ*, 1997, 315(7123):1641

HHR4 Levine, Glenn N., et al. "Pet Ownership and Cardiovascular Risk." *Circulation*, v. 127, n. 23, 9 May 2013. doi:10.1161/CIR.0b013e31829201e1

HHR5 "The Power of Pets. Health Benefits of Human-Animal Interactions." *National Institute of Health, News In Health*, February 2018, newsinhealth.nih.gov/2018/02/power-pets. Accessed 3 February 2020.

HHR6 "Pet care improves youths' diabetes management." *UT Southwestern Medical Center*, 1 November 2015, utswmed.org/medblog/pet-care-youth-diabetes. Accessed 3 February 2020.

Be Purposeful and Service-Oriented

PSO1 Deschene, Lori. "20 Ways to Give Without Expectations." *Tiny Buddha*, tinybuddha.com/blog/20-ways-to-give-without-expectations. Accessed 3 February 2020.

PSO2 Franzen, Alexandra. "50 ways to be ridiculously generous – and feel ridiculously good." *Alexandra Franzen*, 5 September 2013. www.alexandrafranzen.com/2013/09/05/50-ways-to-be-ridiculously-generous. Accessed 3 February 2020.

PSO3 Frey, Thomas. *Epiphany Z: Eight Radical Visions for Transforming Your Future*. New York, NY. Morgan James Publishing. 2017.

PSO4 Walker, Taryn. "Blood donor hits 70-gallon mark." *Colorado Community Media*, 20 July 2015, coloradocommunitymedia.com/stories/blood-donor-hits-70-gallon-mark,193914. Accessed 3 February 2020.

Be Happy and Present

BHP1 Moskowitz, J.T., Epel, E.S., and Acree M. "Positive affect uniquely predicts lower risk of mortality in people with diabetes." *Health Psychology*, 2008 Jan;27(1S):S73-82. doi: 10.1037/0278-6133.27.1.S73.

BHP2 Cohen, Shelden, et al. "Positive Emotional Style Predicts Resistance to Illness After Experimental Exposure to Rhinovirus or Influenza A Virus." *Psychosomatic Medicine*, 68:809 – 815 (2006). doi: 0.1097/01.psy.0000245867.92364.3c.

BHP3 Tindle, Hilary A., et al. "Optimism, Cynical Hostility, and Incident Coronary Heart Disease and Mortality in the Women's Health Initiative." *Circulation*, 2009;120:656–662. doi: 10.1161/CIRCULATIONAHA.108.827642.

BHP4 Lee, Lewina O., et al. "Optimism is associated with exceptional longevity in 2 epidemiologic cohorts of men and women." *Proceedings of the National Academy of Sciences*, Sep 2019, 116 (37) 18357-18362. doi: 10.1073/pnas.1900712116.

BHP5 Baruth, Meghan, et al. "Emotional Outlook on Life Predicts Increases in Physical Activity Among Initially Inactive Men." *Health Education & Behavior*, vol. 38, no. 2, Apr. 2011, pp. 150–158. doi:10.1177/1090198110376352.

BHP6 Mack, Eric. "The Exact Amount of Money it Takes to Make a Person Happy Just Got an Update." *Inc.*, 16 February 2018. www.inc.com/eric-mack/the-exact-amount-of-money-it-takes-to-make-a-person-happy-just-got-an-update.html. Accessed 4 February 2020.

BHP7 Spector, Nicole. "Smiling can trick your brain into happiness – and boost your health." NBC News, 28 November 2017, www.nbcnews.com/better/health/smiling-can-trick-your-brain-happiness-boost-your-health-ncna822591. Accessed 4 February 2020.

BHP8 Tuttle, Dave. "Jack LaLanne." *Life Extension Foundation*, August 2006, www.lifeextension.com/magazine/2006/8/report_lalan ne/page-01. Accessed 4 February 2020.

Use Aesthetics to Feel Better and Live Longer

AFB1 Castle, David J., et al. "Does cosmetic surgery improve psychosocial wellbeing?." *The Medical Journal of Australia*, vol. 176,12 (2002): 601-4.

AFB2 Margraf, Jürgen, et al. "Well-Being From the Knife? Psychological Effects of Aesthetic Surgery." *Clinical Psychological Science*, vol. 1, no. 3, July 2013, pp. 239–252. doi: 10.1177/2167702612471660.

AFB3 Sherman, Neil. "Get A Facelift, Live Longer." *HealthDayNews*, 31 July 2001, consumer.healthday.com/senior-citizen-information-31/misc-aging-news-10/get-a-facelift-live-longer-400737.html. Accessed 4 February 2020.

AFB4 Kader Mohiuddin, Abdul. "Skin Aging & Modern Age Anti-aging Strategies." *Global Journal of Medical Research* [Online], (2019): n. pag. Web. Accessed 4 Feb. 2020.

AFB5 "Ultraviolet (UV) Radiation. What is UV radiation?" *American Cancer Society*, 10 July 2019, www.cancer.org/cancer/cancer-causes/radiation-exposure/uv-radiation.html. Accessed 4 February 2020.

AFB6 Tschinkel, Arielle. "Here's how a vitamin D deficiency might affect your skin." *Insider*, 29 January 2019, www.insider.com/how-does-vitamin-d-affect-your-skin-2019-1#there-are-several-ways-that-being-vitamin-d-deficient-might-impact-your-skin-3. Accessed 4 February 2020.

Have a Health Plan

HP1 Prince, Russ Alan. "The Rise Of Concierge Medical Practices." Forbes, 1 August 2018, www.forbes.com/sites/russalanprince/2018/08/01/the-rise-of-concierge-medical-practices/#1ecc9a14e874. Accessed 4 February 2020.

HP2 Doshi, MD, Sangita. "Your Annual Physical and Why It's Important." *Virtua Health*, 18 December 2019, www.virtua.org/articles/your-annual-physical-and-why-its-important. Accessed 4 February 2020.

HP3 Krans, Brian and Wu, Brian. "Physical Examination." *Healthline*, Medically reviewed by Gregory Minnis 27 June 2017, www.healthline.com/health/physical-examination. Accessed 4 February 2020.

HP4 Roth, Bryan. "Should You Get an Annual Physical?" *Duke Health*, 9 September 2019, www.dukehealth.org/blog/should-you-get-annual-physical. Accessed 4 February 2020.

HP5 "Lab Testing Services." *Life Extension Foundation*, www.lifeextension.com/Vitamins-Supplements/Blood-Tests/Blood-Tests. Accessed 4 February 2020.

HP6 Anderson, James G. and Abrahamson, Kathleen. "Your Health Care May Kill You: Medical Errors." *IOS Press*, vol. 234. doi: 10.3233/978-1-61499-742-9-13.

HP7 "Leading Causes of Death." *CDC/National Center for Health Statistics*, 17 March 2017, www.cdc.gov/nchs/fastats/leading-causes-of-death.htm. Accessed 4 February 2020.

Eat a Natural Diet

END1 Crichton-Stuart, Cathleen. "What are the benefits of eating healthy?" *Medical News Today*, Reviewed 26 June 2018, www.medicalnewstoday.com/articles/322268.php. Accessed 8 February 2020.

END2 Brito, Janet. "5 Foods to Eat for Better Sex – and 3 You Should Really Avoid." *Healthline*, Reviewed 19 June 2018, www.healthline.com/health/food-nutrition/foods-for-better-sex#1. Accessed 8 February 2020.

END3 Katz, D.L. and Meller, S. "Can We Say What Diet Is Best for Health?" *Annual Review of Public Health,* 2014 35:1, 83-103.

END4 Gunnars, Kris. "Protein Intake – How Much Protein Should You Eat Per Day?" *Healthline*, 5 July 2018, www.healthline.com/nutrition/how-much-protein-per-day. Accessed 4 February 2020.

END5 Nowson, Caryl and O'Connell, Stella. "Protein Requirements and Recommendations for Older People: A Review." *Nutrients,* vol. 7,8 6874-99. 14 Aug. 2015. doi:10.3390/nu7085311.

END6 MacAskill, William. "Vegetarians live longer, but it's not because they don't eat meat." *Quartz*, 5 June 2013, qz.com/91123/vegetarians-live-longer-but-its-not-because-they-dont-eat-meat. Accessed 2 February 2020.

END7 Gunnars, Kris. "Intermittent Fasting May Extend Your Lifespan, Helping You Live Longer." *Healthline*, 16 August 2016, healthline.com/nutrition/10-health-benefits-of-intermittent-fasting#section10. Accessed 4 February 2020.

END8 "Doctors need nutrition education, says commentary in JAMA Internal Medicine." *EurekAlert*, 2 July 2019, www.eurekalert.org/pub_releases/2019-07/pcfr-dnn070219.php. Accessed 4 February 2020.

END9 Barnard, N.D. "Ignorance of Nutrition Is No Longer Defensible" *JAMA* Intern Med. 2019, 179(8):1021–1022. doi:10.1001/jamainternmed.2019.2273.

Consider Taking Basic Supplements

SUP1 "Dirt Poor: Have Fruits and Vegetables Become Less Nutritious?" *Scientific American*, 27 April 2011, www.scientificamerican.com/article/soil-depletion-and-nutrition-loss. Accessed 4 February 2020.

SUP2 "Should You Take Dietary Supplements? A Look at Vitamins, Minerals, Botanicals and More." *NIH News in Health*, August 2013, newsinhealth.nih.gov/2013/08/should-you-take-dietary-supplements. Accessed 4 February 2020.

SUP3 Lemon, Jennifer A., et al. "A Complex Dietary Supplement Extends Longevity of Mice." *The Journals of Gerontology*, Series A, Volume 60, Issue 3, March 2005, 275–279. doi: 10.1093/gerona/60.3.275.

SUP4 "Dietary Supplement Health and Education Act of 1994, Public Law 103-417, 103rd Congress." *NIH National Institutes of Health*, 25 October 1994,

ods.od.nih.gov/About/DSHEA_Wording.aspx.
Accessed 4 February 2020.

SUP5 Kresser, Chris. "Well Fed but Undernourished: An American Epidemic." *Kresser Institute*, 28 April 2018, kresserinstitute.com/well-fed-but-undernourished-an-american-epidemic. Accessed 4 February 2020.

SUP6 Bird, Julia K., et al. "Risk of Deficiency in Multiple Concurrent Micronutrients in Children and Adults in the United States." *Nutrients,* vol. 9,7 655. 24 June 2017. doi:10.3390/nu9070655.

SUP7 "Vegetarian and Vegan Diets Explained." *WebMD,* Reviewed by Christine Mikstas, 16 May 2018, www.webmd.com/food-recipes/guide/vegetarian-and-vegan-diet#1. Accessed 4 February 2020.

SUP8 Palsdottir, Hrefna. "Who should take a multivitamin?" *Healthline,* 18 July 2019, www.healthline.com/nutrition/do-multivitamins-work#recommendation. Accessed 4 February 2020.

SUP9 Ware, Megan. "What are the health benefits of vitamin D?" *Medical News Today,* 7 November 2019, www.medicalnewstoday.com/articles/161618.php. Accessed 4 February 2020.

SUP10 Robertson, Ruairi. "13 Benefits of Taking Fish Oil." *Healthline,* 18 December 2018, www.healthline.com/nutrition/13-benefits-of-fish-oil. Accessed 4 February 2020.

SUP11 "Minerals for Bone Health." *American Bone Health,* 28 September 2016, americanbonehealth.org/nutrition/minerals-for-bone-health. Accessed 4 February 2020.

SUP12 Semeco, Arlene. "9 Benefits of Coenzyme Q10 (CoQ10)." *Healthline*, 12 October 2017, www.healthline.com/nutrition/coenzyme-q10. Accessed 4 February 2020.

SUP13 Link, Rachael. "5 Promising Benefits and Uses of Saw Palmetto." *Healthline*, 19 March 2019, www.healthline.com/nutrition/saw-palmetto-benefits. Accessed 4 February 2020.

SUP14 Hill, Ansley. "Does Glucosamine Work? Benefits, Dosage and Side Effects." *Healthline*, 26 September 2018, www.healthline.com/nutrition/glucosamine. Accessed 4 February 2020.

SUP15 Goldschein, Susan. "NAD+ Promotes Stem Cell Renewal and Regenerates Mitochondria." *Life Extension Foundation*, February 2020, www.lifeextension.com/magazine/2020/2/renew-your-own-stem-cells. Accessed 4 February 2020.

SUP16 "Acetyl-L-Carnitine." *WebMD*, www.webmd.com/vitamins/ai/ingredientmono-834/acetyl-l-carnitine. Accessed 4 February 2020.

SUP17 Castro, M. Regina. "Diabetes treatment: Can cinnamon lower blood sugar?" *Mayo Clinic*, www.mayoclinic.org/diseases-conditions/diabetes/expert-answers/diabetes/faq-20058472. Accessed 4 February 2020.

Move Your Body

MYB1 Rieck, Thom. "10,000 steps a day: Too low? Too high?" *Mayo Clinic*, 16 March 2018, www.mayoclinic.org/healthy-lifestyle/fitness/in-depth/10000-steps/art-20317391. Accessed 5 February 2020.

MYB2 "Physical Activity – Current Guidelines." ODPHP *Office of Disease Prevention and Health Promotion,* health.gov/paguidelines/second-edition. Accessed 5 February 2020.

MYB3 "Benefits of Exercise." *MedlinePlus,* medlineplus.gov/benefitsofexercise.html. Accessed 5 February 2020.

MYB4 "US Half Marathon Race Results." *Athlinks,* 6 June 2004, www.athlinks.com/event/49692/results/Event/2502/Course/3991/Bib/327. Accessed 5 February 2020.

MYB5 "2015 NPC Teen Collegiate & Masters National Championships." *NPC News Online,* 15 July 2015, contests.npcnewsonline.com/contests/2015/npc_teen_collegiate__masters_national_championships. Accessed 5 February 2020.

MYB6 "Bantam Weight Comparison Pictures." *NPC News Online,* Greg Damian second from right stage right, contests.npcnewsonline.com/images.php?image=1354098&contest=2015%20NPC%20Teen%20Collegiate%20&%20Masters%20National%20Championships&title=Comparisons%20&ids=1354071,1354074,1354077,1354080,1354082,1354085,1354088,1354090,1354093,1354095,1354098,1354101,1354104,1354107. Accessed 5 February 2020.

MYB7 "Running Heart Rate Zones | The Basics." *Polar,* 19 April 2016, updated 21 February 2020, www.polar.com/blog/running-heart-rate-zones-basics. Accessed 5 February 2020.

MYB8 Stull, Kyle. "Built to Order: Strength and Size Require Different Approaches." *American Fitness Magazine*, Fall 2017, magazine.nasm.org/american-fitness-magazine/issues/american-fitness-magazine-fall-2017/built-to-order-strength-and-size-require-different-approaches. Accessed 5 February 2020.

Maintain Healthy Body Composition

HBC1 Ilavskáa, Silvia, et al. "Association between the human immune response and body mass index." *Human Immunology*, Vol. 73, Issue 5, May 2012, Pages 480-485. doi: 10.1016/j.humimm.2012.02.023.

HBC2 Soleymani, MD, Taraneh. "Can My Weight Cause Memory Issues?" *OAC Obesity Action Coalition*, Summer 2017, https://www.obesityaction.org/community/article-library/can-my-weight-cause-memory-issues/. Accessed 7 February 2020.

HBC3 Allison, D.B., et al. "Annual Deaths Attributable to Obesity in the United States." *JAMA*. 1999, 282(16):1530–1538. doi: 10.1001/jama.282.16.1530.

HBC4 Hales, Craig M., et al. "Prevalence of Obesity Among Adults and Youth: United States, 2015-2016." *Centers for Disease Control, Prevention National Center for Health Statistics*, October 2017, www.cdc.gov/nchs/data/databriefs/db288.pdf, Accessed 5 February 2020.

HBC5 Brazier, Yvette. "How useful is body mass index (BMI)?" *Medical News Today*, Reviewed 16 August 2017., www.medicalnewstoday.com/articles/255712.php. Accessed 5 February 2020.

HBC6 "Calculate Your Body Mass Index." *NIH National Heart, Lung, and Blood Institute,* www.nhlbi.nih.gov/health/educational/lose_wt/BMI/bmicalc.htm. Accessed 5 February 2020.

HBC7 "About Adult BMI." *CDC Centers for Disease Control and Prevention,* Division of Nutrition, Physical Activity, and Obesity, National Center for Chronic Disease Prevention and Health Promotion, 29 August 2017, www.cdc.gov/healthyweight/assessing/bmi/adult_bm i/index.html. Accessed 5 February 2020.

HBC8 DuVall, Jeremey. "The 5 Best Ways to Measure Body Fat Percentage." *Health.com,* 12 August 2014, www.health.com/fitness/the-5-best-ways-to-measure-body-fat-percentage. Accessed 5 February 2020.

HBC9 Muth, Natalie Digate. "What are the guidelines for percentage of body fat loss?" *ACE American Council on Exercise,* 2 December 2009, www.acefitness.org/education-and-resources/lifestyle/blog/112/what-are-the-guidelines-for-percentage-of-body-fat-loss. Accessed 5 February 2020.

Optimize Your Hormones

OYH1 "Endocrinology & Diabetes Research." *SciTechnol,* www.scitechnol.com/endocrinology-and-diabetes-research.php. Accessed 5 February 2020.

OYH2 Brown-Borg, Holly M. "Hormonal regulation of longevity in mammals." *Ageing research reviews* vol. 6,1 (2007): 28-45. doi:10.1016/j.arr.2007.02.005.

OYH3 Decaroli, Maria Chiara, and Vincenzo Rochira. "Aging and sex hormones in males." *Virulence,* vol. 8,5 (2017): 545-570. doi:10.1080/21505594.2016.1259053.

OYH4 Gotter, Ana, et al. "Low Testosterone in Men." *Healthline,* Reviewed 27 February 2019, www.healthline.com/health/side-effects-of-low-testosterone. Accessed 5 February 2020.

OYH5 Boyle, P., et al. "Endogenous and exogenous testosterone and the risk of prostate cancer and increased prostate-specific antigen (PSA) level: a meta-analysis." *BJU Int,* 2016 Nov;118(5):731-741. doi: 10.1111/bju.13417.

OYH6 "Hormone Therapy to Treat Cancer." *NIH National Cancer Institute,* 29 April 2015, www.cancer.gov/about-cancer/treatment/types/hormone-therapy. Accessed 5 February 2020.

OYH7 Cherney, Kristeen. "Effects of Menopause on the Body." *Healthline,* Reviewed 5 February 2019, www.healthline.com/health/menopause/hrt-effects-on-body#1. Accessed 5 February 2020.

OYH8 Compounding and the FDA: Questions and Answers." *U.S. Food and Drug Administration,* 21 June 2018, www.fda.gov/drugs/human-drug-compounding/compounding-and-fda-questions-and-answers. Accessed 6 February 2020.

OYH9 Writing Group for the Women's Health Initiative Investigators. "Risks and Benefits of Estrogen Plus Progestin in Healthy Postmenopausal Women: Principal Results From the Women's Health Initiative Randomized Controlled Trial." *JAMA.* 2002;288(3):321–333. doi: 10.1001/jama.288.3.321.

OYH10 Files, Julia A., et al. "Bioidentical hormone therapy." *Mayo Clinic Proceedings,* vol. 86,7 (2011): 673-80, quiz 680. doi:10.4065/mcp.2010.0714.

OYH11 Kannegaard, P.N., et al. "Excess mortality in men compared with women following a hip fracture. National analysis of comedications, comorbidity and survival." *Age Ageing.* 2010 Mar;39(2):203-9. doi: 10.1093/ageing/afp221. Epub 14 Jan 2010.

OYH12 Faloon, William, "Misguided Medicine." *Life Extension Magazine,* June 2014, www.lifeextension.com/magazine/2014/6/misguided-medicine/page-01. Accessed 5 February 2020.

OYH13 Barry, Daniel W., Gerlach, Amanda, Damian, Greg and Kohrt, Wendy M. "Bone Density – Triathlete." *Medicine & Science in Sports & Exercise:* May 2007, Vol. 39, I. 5, p. S106. doi: 10.1249/01.mss.0000273339.18490.55.

Avoid Toxic Substances

ATS1 "Metabolic Detoxification." *Life Extension Magazine,* www.lifeextension.com/protocols/metabolic-health/metabolic-detoxification/page-07. Accessed 7 February 2020.

ATS2 Spritzler, Franziska. "7 'Toxins' in Food That Are Actually Concerning." *Healthline,* 23 May 2016, www.healthline.com/nutrition/7-food-toxins-that-are-concerning. Accessed 7 February 2020.

ATS3 The American Cancer Society medical and editorial content team. "Harmful Chemicals in Tobacco Products." *American Cancer Society,* 5 April 2017, www.cancer.org/cancer/cancer-causes/tobacco-and-cancer/carcinogens-found-in-tobacco-products.html. Accessed 7 February 2020.

ATS4 "Electronic Smoking Devices and Secondhand Aerosol." *ANRF American Nonsmokers' Rights Foundation*, 2019, no-smoke.org/electronic-smoking-devices-secondhand-aerosol. Accessed 7 February 2020.

ATS5 Hughes, Locke. "How Does Too Much Sugar Affect Your Body." *WebMD*, Reviewed by Nazario, Brunilda 17 December 2019, www.webmd.com/diabetes/features/how-sugar-affects-your-body. Accessed 7 February 2020.

ATS6 "10 Reasons Why Sugar Is Bad for Your Health." *Atkins*, www.atkins.com/how-it-works/library/articles/10-ways-sugar-harms-your-health. Accessed 7 February 2020.

ATS7 Gunnars, Kris. "Is Fructose Bad for You? The Surprising Truth." *Healthline*, 23 April 2018, www.healthline.com/nutrition/why-is-fructose-bad-for-you. Accessed 7 February 2020.

ATS8 "Added Sugars." *American Heart Association*, Last Reviewed, 17 April 2018, www.heart.org/en/healthy-living/healthy-eating/eat-smart/sugar/added-sugars. Accessed 7 February 2020.

ATS9 "Dietary Guidelines for Americans. 2015-2020." *U.S. Department of Agriculture*, December 2015, health.gov/dietaryguidelines/2015/resources/2015-2020_Dietary_Guidelines.pdf. Accessed 7 February 2020.

ATS10 "Taking the Trans Fat Out. Banning Trans Fats in Schools, Workplaces, and Restaurants." American Heart Association, 2015, www.heart.org/idc/groups/heart-public/@wcm/@adv/documents/downloadable/ucm_4 80245.pdf. Accessed 7 February 2020.

ATS11 "The FDA CLARITY Study." *Facts About BPA, Polycarbonate/BPA Global Group*, 28 September 2018, www.factsaboutbpa.org/scientific-assessments/fda-clarity-study?gclid=Cj0KCQjwoKzsBRC5ARIsAITcwXHv0XKB 3agvX1Ek1-7qTp2MvkSE0IheN7qpiFVeEC8NYtediD9VMrcaAtJfEA Lw_wcB. Accessed 7 February 2020.

ATS12 vom Saal, Frederick S., et al. "Chapel Hill bisphenol A expert panel consensus statement: integration of mechanisms, effects in animals and potential to impact human health at current levels of exposure." *Reproductive Toxicology (Elmsford, N.Y.)*, vol. 24,2 (2007): 131-8. doi:10.1016/j.reprotox.2007.07.005.

ATS13 Davis, Charles Patrick. "Mercury Poisoning" *eMedicineHealth.com*, Reviewed 14 November 2019, www.emedicinehealth.com/mercury_poisoning/article_ em.htm. Accessed 7 February 2020.

ATS14 "Tony Robbins attributes Quicksilver Scientific® to lower Mercury Levels." *Prnewswire.com/news/Quicksilver-Scientific*, 10 September 2018, www.prnewswire.com/news-releases/tony-robbins-attributes-quicksilver-scientific-to-lower-mercury-levels-300709178.html. Accessed 7 February 2020.

ATS15 Wani, Ab Latif, et al. "Lead toxicity: a review." *Interdisciplinary Toxicology*, vol. 8,2 (2015): 55-64. doi:10.1515/intox-2015-0009.

ATS16 Baan, Robert, et al. "Carcinogenicity of alcoholic beverages." *The Lancet, Oncology,* vol. 8,4 (2007): 292-3. doi:10.1016/s1470-2045(07)70099-2.

ATS17 *Global status report on alcohol and health.* WHO Press, Geneva, Switzerland, 2011.

ATS18 "Cinnamon: The Good, the Bad, and the Tasty." *GI Society, Canadian Society of Intestinal Research,* 2017, badgut.org/information-centre/health-nutrition/cinnamon. Accessed 7 February 2020.

Protect Your Brain

PYB1 "2018 Alzheimer's Disease Facts and Figures." *Alzheimer's Association,* 2018, www.alz.org/media/documents/facts-and-figures-2018-r.pdf. Accessed 7 February 2020.

PYB2 Holland, Kimberly. "What Are the 12 Leading Causes of Death in the United States? 6. Alzheimer's disease." *Healthline,* Reviewed 1 November 2018, www.healthline.com/health/leading-causes-of-death#alzheimers-disease. Accessed 7 February 2020.

PYB3 Mayo Clinic Staff. "Alzheimer's treatments: What's on the horizon?" *Mayo Clinic,* 19 April 2019, www.mayoclinic.org/diseases-conditions/alzheimers-disease/in-depth/alzheimers-treatments/art-20047780. Accessed 7 February 2020.

PYB4 DeClaire, Joan. "7 ways to protect your brain—and your thinking power." *Kaiser Permanente Washington Health Research Institute,* 3 September 2015, www.kpwashingtonresearch.org/live-healthy/all-articles/live-healthy-2015/7-ways-protect-your-brain-and-your-thinking-power. Accessed 7 February 2020.

PYB5 Sabia, Séverine, et al. "Impact of smoking on cognitive decline in early old age: the Whitehall II cohort study." *Archives of general psychiatry*, vol. 69,6 (2012): 627-35. doi:10.1001/archgenpsychiatry.2011.2016.

PYB6 Rehfeld, Kathrin, et al. "Dancing or Fitness Sport? The Effects of Two Training Programs on Hippocampal Plasticity and Balance Abilities in Healthy Seniors." *Frontiers in Human Neuroscience*, 11:305. doi: 10.3389/fnhum.2017.00305.

PYB7 Bratman, Gregory N., et al. "Nature reduces rumination and sgPFC activation." *Proceedings of the National Academy of Sciences*, July 2015, 112 (28) 8567-8572. doi: 10.1073/pnas.1510459112.

PYB8 Firth, Joseph, et al. "The Effects of Dietary Improvement on Symptoms of Depression and Anxiety: A Meta-Analysis of Randomized Controlled Trials." *Psychosomatic Medicine*, vol. 81,3 (2019): 265-280. doi:10.1097/PSY.0000000000000673.

PYB9 "Mushrooms may reduce risk of cognitive decline." *NUS [National University of Singapore] News*, 12 March 2019, news.nus.edu.sg/research/mushrooms-reduce-cognitive-decline. Accessed 7 February 2020.

PYB10 West, Helen. "The 10 Best Nootropic Supplements to Boost Brain Power. #3 Caffeine." *Healthline*, 26 November 2016, www.healthline.com/nutrition/best-nootropic-brain-supplements#section3. Accessed 7 February 2020.

PYB11 Stonehouse, Welma, et al. "DHA supplementation improved both memory and reaction time in healthy young adults: a randomized controlled trial." *The American Journal of Clinical Nutrition,* vol. 97,5 (2013): 1134-43. doi:10.3945/ajcn.112.053371.

PYB12 Martins, Julian G. "EPA but not DHA appears to be responsible for the efficacy of omega-3 long chain polyunsaturated fatty acid supplementation in depression: evidence from a meta-analysis of randomized controlled trials." *Journal of the American College of Nutrition,* vol. 28,5 (2009): 525-42. doi:10.1080/07315724.2009.10719785.

PYB13 Curtin, Melanie. "50-year-olds can have the brains of 25-year-olds if they meditate, memory and decision-making research shows." *Business Insider,* 21 February 2020, www.businessinsider.com/neuroscience-50-year-olds-brains-of-25-year-olds-habit-2019-4. Accessed 7 February 2020.

PYB14 Hölzel, Britta K., et al. "Mindfulness practice leads to increases in regional brain gray matter density." *Psychiatry Research,* vol. 191,1 (2011): 36-43. doi:10.1016/j.pscychresns.2010.08.006.

PYB15 Herrmann, Ned. "What is the function of the various brainwaves?" *Scientific American,* 22 December 1997, www.scientificamerican.com/article/what-is-the-function-of-t-1997-12-22.

PYB16 "Brain training built on science." *Lumosity,* www.lumosity.com/en/science. Accessed 7 February 2020.

Choose the Right Amount of Stress

STR1 Yaribeygi, Habib, et al. "The impact of stress on body function: A review." *EXCLI Journal,* vol. 16 1057-1072. 21 July 2017. doi:10.17179/excli2017-480.

STR2 Higuera, Valencia. "What Is General Adaptation Syndrome?" *Healthline*, Reviewed 1 May 2017, www.healthline.com/health/general-adaptation-syndrome. Accessed 7 February 2020.

STR3 Thompson, Alexandra. "Can Stress Kill You?" The American Institute of Stress, 8 November, 2019, https://www.stress.org/can-stress-kill-you. Accessed 25 April 2020.

STR4 Scott, Elizabeth. "Effective Stress Relievers for Your Life." *Verywell Mind*, Updated on 8 January 2020, www.verywellmind.com/tips-to-reduce-stress-3145195. Accessed 7 February 2020.

STR5 Jennings, Kerri-Ann. "16 Simple Ways to Relieve Stress and Anxiety." *Healthline*, 28 August 2018, www.healthline.com/nutrition/16-ways-relieve-stress-anxiety. Accessed 7 February 2020.

STR6 Mayo Clinic Staff. "Relaxation techniques: Try these steps to reduce stress." *Mayo Clinic*, 19 April 2017, www.mayoclinic.org/healthy-lifestyle/stress-management/in-depth/relaxation-technique/art-20045368. Accessed 7 February 2020.

STR7 "Stress is a normal reaction the body has when changes occur. It can respond to these changes physically, mentally, or emotionally." *Cleveland Clinic*, Reviewed 5 February 2015, my.clevelandclinic.org/health/articles/11874-stress.

STR8 Kress, MD, Anna. "3 Steps to Releasing Your Attachment to an Outcome." *Dr. Anna Kress*, 5 February 2019, drannakress.com/3-steps-to-releasing-your-attachment-to-an-outcome. Accessed 7 February 2020.

References

Sleep Seven Hours Per Night

SL1 Smith, Yolanda. "Function of Sleep." *News Medical Life Sciences*, 23 August 2018, www.news-medical.net/health/Function-of-Sleep.aspx. Accessed 7 February 2020.

SL2 "Sleep loss limits fat loss, study finds." *UChicago News*, 4 October 2010, news.uchicago.edu/story/sleep-loss-limits-fat-loss-study-finds. Accessed 7 February 2020.

SL3 Xie, LuLu, et al. "Sleep Drives Metabolite Clearance from the Adult Brain." *Science*, 18 October 2013: Vol. 342, Issue 6156, pp. 373-377. doi: 10.1126/science.1241224.

SL4 Nagai, Michiaki, et al. "Sleep duration as a risk factor for cardiovascular disease – a review of the recent literature." *Current Cardiology Reviews,* vol. 6,1 (2010): 54-61. doi:10.2174/157340310790231635.

SL5 Covassin, Naima, and Singh, Prachi. "Sleep Duration and Cardiovascular Disease Risk: Epidemiologic and Experimental Evidence." *Sleep Medicine Clinics* vol. 11,1 (2016): 81-9. doi:10.1016/j.jsmc.2015.10.007.

SL6 DiGiulio, Sarah. "What Happens in Your Body and Brain While You Sleep." *NBC News/Better*, 9 October 2017, www.nbcnews.com/better/health/what-happens-your-body-brain-while-you-sleep-ncna805276. Accessed 7 February 2020.

SL7 Kripke, Daniel F., et al. "Mortality associated with sleep duration and insomnia." *Archives of General Psychiatry,* vol. 59,2 (2002): 131-6. doi:10.1001/archpsyc.59.2.131.

SL8 Kripke, Daniel F., et al. "Mortality related to actigraphic long and short sleep." Sleep Medicine, vol. 12,1 (2011): 28-33. doi:10.1016/j.sleep.2010.04.016.

SL9 "Understanding Sleep Cycles: What Happens While You Sleep." *National Sleep Foundation*, www.sleep.org/articles/what-happens-during-sleep. Accessed 7 February 2020.

SL10 Mozes, Alan. "Poor REM Sleep, Higher Risk for Depression?" *WebMD*, 8 February 2016, www.webmd.com/depression/news/20160208/poor-rem-sleep-may-be-linked-to-higher-risk-for-anxiety-depression#1. Accessed 7 February 2020.

SL11 "REM Sleep and Our Dreaming Lives." *S+ResMed*, sleep.mysplus.com/library/category3/REM_Sleep_and_Our_Dreaming_Lives.html. Accessed 7 February 2020.

SL12 Brown, G. M. "Light, melatonin and the sleep-wake cycle." *Journal of Psychiatry & Neuroscience: JPN*, vol. 19,5 (1994): 345-53.

SL13 Khullar, MD, Atul. "The Role of Melatonin in the Circadian Rhythm Sleep-Wake Cycle." *MJH Life Sciences Psychiatric Times*, 10 July 2012, www.psychiatrictimes.com/sleep-disorders/role-melatonin-circadian-rhythm-sleep-wake-cycle. Accessed 7 February 2020.

SL14 Reiter, Russel J., et al. "Melatonin as an antioxidant: under promises but over delivers." *Journal of Pineal Research*, vol. 61,3 (2016): 253-78. doi:10.1111/jpi.12360.

SL15 Karasek, M. "Melatonin, human aging, and age-related diseases." *Experimental Gerontology*, vol. 39,11-12 (2004): 1723-9. doi:10.1016/j.exger.2004.04.012.

References

SL16 "Healthy Sleep Tips." *National Sleep Foundation*, www.sleepfoundation.org/articles/healthy-sleep-tips. Accessed 7 February 2020.

Conclusion of the Longevity Best Practices

CLB1 Rollins, Jarod, et al. "Synergistic Cellular Pathways Identified That Extend Lifespan by 500%." SciTechDaily, 5 February 2020, scitechdaily.com/synergistic-cellular-pathways-identified-that-extend-lifespan-by-500. Accessed 8 February 2020.

Advanced Anti-Aging Techniques

PC1 Foroutan, Behzad. "Personalized Medicine: A Review with Regard to Biomarkers." *Journal of Bioequivalence & Bioavailability*, 2015, 7:6. doi: 10.4172/jbb.1000248.

PC2 *PMC Personalized Medicine Coalition*, www.personalizedmedicinecoalition.org. Accessed 8 February 2020.

PC3 Walter, Zuzanna. "Personalized Nutrition Science for Optimal Health." *American Academy of Anti-Aging Medicine*, 9 August 2019, blog.a4m.com/personalized-nutrition-science-for-optimal-health. Accessed 8 February 2020.

PRP1 "Platelet-Rich Plasma (PRP) Injections." *HSS Hospital for Special Surgery*, www.hss.edu/condition-list_prp-injections.asp. Accessed 8 February 2020.

PRP2 Cafasso, Jacquelyn. "Stem Cell Research." *Healthline*, Reviewed 6 April 2016, www.healthline.com/health/stem-cell-research. Accessed 8 February 2020.

PRP3 "Stem Cell Information." *NIH National Institutes of Health*, stemcells.nih.gov/info/basics/1.htm. Accessed 8 February 2020.

PRP4 "Bone Marrow Stem Cell Transplant – HSCT." *MS National Multiple Sclerosis Society*, www.nationalmssociety.org/Research/Research-News-Progress/Stem-Cells-in-MS/Bone-Marrow-Stem-Cell-Transplant-%E2%80%93-HSCT. Accessed 8 February 2020.

DS1 Klimova, Blanka, et al. "Anti-Aging Drugs – Prospect of Longer Life?" *Current Medicinal Chemistry*, Vol. 25, I. 17, 2018. doi: 10.2174/0929867325666171129215251.

DS2 Blagosklonny, M.V. "Rapamycin for longevity: opinion article." *Aging*, 2019, 11:8048-8067. doi: 10.18632/aging.102355.

DS3 "Senolytic Therapies to Clear Senescent Cells will Transform the Field of Medicine for Age-Related Conditions." *Fight Aging!*, 5 September 2017, www.fightaging.org/archives/2017/09/senolytic-therapies-to-clear-senescent-cells-will-transform-the-field-of-medicine-for-age-related-conditions. Accessed 8 February 2020.

DS4 "First-in-human trial of senolytic drugs encouraging." *Medical Xpress*, 7 January 2019, medicalxpress.com/news/2019-01-first-in-human-trial-senolytic-drugs.html.

References

DS5 Kirkland, J.L., Tchkonia, T., Zhu, Y., Niedernhofer, L.J., and Robbins, P.D. "The Clinical Potential of Senolytic Drugs." *J Am Geriatr Soc*, 65: 2297-2301. doi: 10.1111/jgs.14969.

DS6 Corbyn, Zoë. "Want to live for ever? Flush out your zombie cells." *The Guardian*, 6 October 2018, www.theguardian.com/science/2018/oct/06/race-to-kill-killer-zombie-cells-senescent-damaged-ageing-eliminate-research-mice-aubrey-de-grey. Accessed 8 February 2020.

OA1 Zullo, J.M., Drake, D., Aron, L., et al. "Regulation of lifespan by neural excitation and REST." *Nature* 574, 359-364 (2019). doi: 10.1038/s41586-019-1647-8.

OA2 Biegler, Paul. "Brain activity linked to longevity." *Cosmos*, 17 October 2019, cosmosmagazine.com/biology/brain-activity-linked-to-longevity. Accessed 8 February 2020.

OA3 Zullo, J.M., Drake, D., Aron, L., et al. "Regulation of lifespan by neural excitation and REST." *Nature* 574, 359-364 (2019). doi: 10.1038/s41586-019-1647-8.

OA4 Hayasaki, Erika. "Has this scientist finally found the fountain of youth." MIT Technology Review, 8 August 2019, www.technologyreview.com/s/614074/scientist-fountain-of-youth-epigenome. Accessed 8 February 2020.

OA5 Brownell, Lindsay. "A swifter way towards 3D-printed organs." *Wyss Institute*, 6 September 2019, www.wyss.harvard.edu/a-swifter-way-towards-3d-printed-organs. Accessed 8 February 2020.

OA6 Gander, Kashmira. "3D-Printed Living Skin with Blood Vessels Created by Scientists." *Newsweek*, 4 November 2019, www.newsweek.com/3d-printed-living-skin-blood-vessels-scientists-1469507. Accessed 8 February 2020.

OA7 Fan, Shelly. "AI Won't Replace Doctors, It Will Augment Them." *Singularity Hub*, 7 November 2018, singularityhub.com/2018/11/07/ai-wont-replace-doctors-it-will-augment-them. Accessed 8 February 2020.

OA8 Kahan, John. "Using AI to advance the health of people and communities around the world." *Microsoft*, 29 January 2020, blogs.microsoft.com/on-the-issues/2020/01/29/ai-for-health-child-mortality. Accessed 8 February 2020.

AG1 de Grey, Aubrey, and Rae, Michael. *Ending Aging: The Rejuvenation Breakthroughs That Could Reverse Human Aging in Our Lifetime*. New York, NY, St. Martin's Press, 2007.

AG2 *Methuselah Foundation*, www.mfoundation.org. Accessed 8 February 2020.

AG3 *Exponential Medicine*, exponential.singularityu.org/medicine/about. Accessed 8 February 2020.

AG4 *Regenerative Medicine Foundation*, www.regmedfoundation.org. Accessed 8 February 2020.

AG5 *American Academy of Anti-Aging Medicine*, www.a4m.com/our-mission.html. Accessed 8 February 2020.

References

AG6 *Fight Aging!*, www.fightaging.org/about/#mission. Accessed 8 February 2020.

Reasons for Hope and Optimism

RHO1 Hyatt, David Graham and Spicer, Andrew. "Walmart tried to make sustainability affordable. Here's what happened." *Quartz at Work*, 13 August 2018, qz.com/work/1354706/walmart-tried-to-make-sustainability-affordable-heres-what-happened. Accessed 7 February 2020.

RHO2 *The Sustainability Consortium*, www.sustainabilityconsortium.org. Accessed 7 February 2020.

RHO3 "One Planet, How Many People? A Review of Earth's Carrying Capacity." *UNEP Global Environmental Alert Service*, June 2012, https://na.unep.net/geas/archive/pdfs/geas_jun_12_c arrying_capacity.pdf. Accessed 7 February 2020.

RHO4 Goldman, Dana. "The Economic Promise of Delayed Aging." *Cold Spring Harbor Perspectives in Medicine*, vol. 6,2 a025072. 18 Dec. 2015. doi:10.1101/cshperspect.a025072.

RHO5 Rifkin, Jeremy. *The Zero Marginal Cost Society*. New York, NY, St. Martin's Press, 2014.

RHO6 Diamandis, Peter. "The Future of Food: 3D Printing, Vertical Farming & Materials Science (Part 1)" *Diamandis*, www.diamandis.com/blog/future-faster-future-of-food-part-1. Accessed 7 February 2020.

RHO7 Diamandis, Peter. "The Future of Food: Protein in 2030 (Part 2)." *Diamandis*, www.diamandis.com/blog/future-faster-future-of-food-part-2. Accessed 7 February 2020.

RHO8 "Annual Global Road Crash Statistics." *ASIRT Association for Safe International Road Travel,* www.asirt.org/safe-travel/road-safety-facts. Accessed 7 February 2020.

RHO9 "Highly automated technologies, often called self-driving cars, promise a range of potential benefits." *Coalition for Future Mobility,* coalitionforfuturemobility.com/benefits-of-self-driving-vehicles. Accessed 7 February 2020.

RHO10 Hymowitz, Carol. "Governments And Employers Need To Get Real About Longevity." *Forbes,* 24 December 2019, www.forbes.com/sites/nextavenue/2019/12/24/gover nments-and-employers-need-to-get-real-about-longevity/#6c39e4bf115e. Accessed 7 February 2020.

Afterword, COVID-19

AC1 "WHO Director-General calls on G20 to Fight, Unite, and Ignite against COVID-19," *World Health Organization,* 26 March 2020, www.who.int/news-room/detail/26-03-2020-who-s-director-general-calls-on-g20-to-fight-unite-and-ignite-against-covid-19?fbclid=IwAR2v1as5sqCXYUxbaLoLtZ73NuLn1kAGG MXtkHoLEShyWGKZIh3CmquzpCE. Accessed 27 March 2020.

Part IX. Epilogue – The Miracle

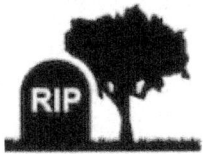

In May of 2019, my father fell and went to the emergency room. The emergency room staff x-rayed his leg, diagnosed him with a broken fibula and released him to see an orthopedic specialist. I was not sure if I wanted to see my father in Alabama. Two years prior, my father recovered from a heart attack. I did not visit him then.

My father and I did not have a good relationship. From what I can tell, he did not have a good relationship with anyone. He did have one dear relationship and that was with alcohol. My father's drinking was functional. He was able to go to work and pay the bills. He had four children, of whom I was the eldest. He was not involved with any of his children. I decided to go to Alabama, mainly because I wanted to support my family.

When I arrived, my father had not been able to get up from his sofa for two days. The broken bone exposed how sick he was. I called 911 to take him back to the hospital. This time, the hospital admitted him. Over the summer and fall, my father moved back and forth between the hospital, nursing care, and his home. I returned several times to Alabama and helped my family and my father with several important tasks.

I did not realize how much my father's behavior had affected me until I went to Alanon meetings. In Alanon, I learned that alcoholism is a family disease. Everyone is affected by a problem drinker. In my trips back to Alabama, I sometimes observed selfish behaviors in my father and I realized I did some of the same things. I thought I had grown past this, but I had not. During an Alanon meeting a few weeks prior to my father's passing, someone shared that he had forgiven his son for all of the problems his son had caused. I immediately asked myself if I could forgive my father and my answer was, "No, I do not think I can." A few minutes later, another person shared that a miracle had happened in her life. I concluded that I was open to the possibility that a miracle could happen and I could forgive my father. That was as close to forgiving him as I could get.

My father hated being in the hospital or a nursing home. In November 2019, he was confined to a skilled care nursing facility for six weeks after a hospital visit because he needed an antibiotic infusion. On Monday, December 9, the infusion cycle was complete. He was excited because he was going to go home. Unfortunately, his health had deteriorated. He could barely walk. He had been evaluated by hospice and they would accept him if he wanted that. He wanted to think about that before agreeing.

My father lived by himself and should not have been home alone. The next morning, my sister went to see him and the situation was dire. He had cut his foot and blood was everywhere. My sister insisted that he could not continue to live alone without support. Considering his options, he agreed to engage hospice.

I almost flew out that day but waited to see if the situation improved. It did not. On Thursday, December 12, my sister and I arrived at my father's house first thing in the morning. The situation had still not improved. My sister pleaded with my father to allow us to take him back to the nursing home. My father's response was dramatic. He threw the covers over his head and said he was not leaving. However, the hospice resources were coming and were beginning to help.

Throughout this day, my father would sometimes be sharp and coherent and at other times he seemed to be moving in and out of consciousness. At one point, he mentioned someone was outside in the backyard. I looked but I did not see anyone.

The hospice nurse arrived late that afternoon and took his vital signs. My father was stable and the nurse left. At that point, I was the only person there with my father. We knew that my father would need additional help, and I had arranged for another nursing assistant to meet my father the next day. I asked him if he would be okay with that. Something happened in that moment that changed everything. He asked me if I would be there. It was a vulnerable moment, the kind of moment we never had before because I had never felt that he needed me. I said, "Yes. I will be there." I asked him if he needed anything else, he said "no", and I left.

The next morning, I found him right where I had left him. He had died in his sleep. There was no struggle. His hands were in his pockets. The irony of all of this is that I was there, not in Denver where I lived. I was the last person to talk with him. I found my father by myself. My brother, who had provided much support for my father, was out of town that week.

That day, I gave the news of my father's passing to my meditation group in Denver. After the group meditation that evening, one of the meditators said that my father had come to her. My father asked her to tell me that he loved me and asked for my forgiveness. The last moment that I had with my father was profound and I had peace. I did not think of any of the other experiences I had with him, only that last one. I had forgiven him. I believe the miracle happened when I became open to the possibility that I might be able to forgive my father.

I gave the eulogy at my father's funeral service. I concluded with, "Dad, I love you and I forgive you."

A couple of weeks after my father died, my mother, who had been divorced from my father for almost 40 years, sent the following text to my brother and sister and me, "I love you, dear family, with all my heart. I love the way you walked with your father through the summer/fall, the last moments of his life. I love you for your care. I know if I am in need, you will be there too. Bless you!

Part X. About the Author

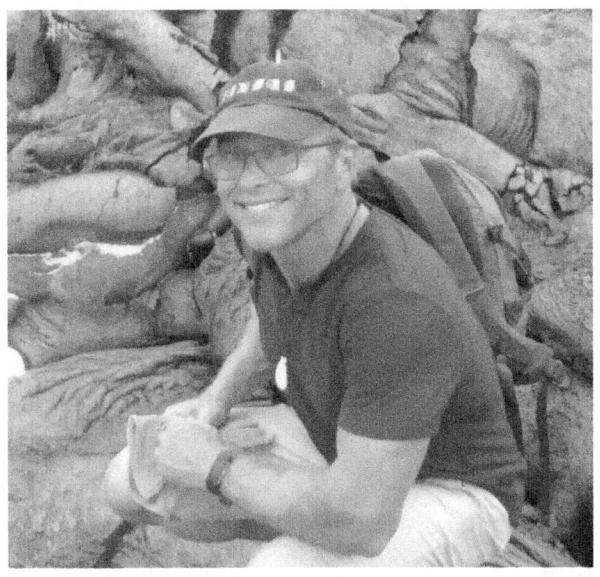

Gregory Robert Damian was born in 1962 in Huntington, IN. In 1983, he received his BS in engineering from the University of Alabama in Huntsville. In 1984, he earned an MSME degree with a focus on robotic technology from the Georgia Institute of Technology. In 1989, he completed his Master's in Business Administration (MBA) from Indiana University with an emphasis on information technology. In 2006, he completed medical school prerequisites and started a biomedical engineering PhD program from which he later withdrew.

He has worked in information technology roles for large international corporations, including Ford, SAP, and Oracle. He is a certified Project Management

Professional (PMP) as well as a certified Scrum Master (CSM).

He is a NASM Certified Personal Trainer (CPT) and has also held the ACE personal trainer certification. He also holds personal training certifications from the Colgan Institute and earned the Certified Sports Nutrition Advisor status from the Cory Holly Institute.

In 1988, he started competing in running and triathlon races. He completed two full marathons, many half marathons, and shorter running races, as well as Half Ironman and shorter distance triathlon races. His best result was winning the US Half Marathon running race in Denver, CO, in 2004. In 2012, he was ranked 217 out of 2,793 male triathletes (top 8%) in the US in the 50-to-54 age group.

In 2004, he performed 495 pull-ups in an hour in a world record attempt. The world record at that time was 504 pull-ups. In his 50s, he won pull-up contests by completing over 40 pull-ups in one set.

He won two Colorado State bantamweight bodybuilding competitions in his 50s and, in 2015, won third place in the Master's men-35-and-over division at the Masters Nationals Bodybuilding event in Pittsburgh, PA.

In 2017, he sold all his belongings and moved to a yoga center on the Big Island of Hawaii. After living and working there for three months, he traveled to Ecuador where he volunteered at a retreat center, studied

Spanish, and visited the Galapagos Islands where he dove with hammerhead sharks.

For work and for pleasure, he has traveled to 49 states in the US and to over 30 countries in Europe, Asia, and Latin America. He owned property in Costa Rica. He studied Japanese and speaks intermediate Spanish.

He currently lives near Denver, CO, and has hiked 20 of Colorado's mountains higher than 14,000 feet. He volunteers for several organizations in the Denver area.

Made in the USA
Monee, IL
14 July 2020